COLOR ATLAS &
SYNOPSIS OF
CLINICAL
OPHTHALMOLOGY

WILLS EYE HOSPITAL

NEURO-
OPHTHALMOLOGY

COLOR ATLAS AND SYNOPSIS OF CLINICAL OPHTHALMOLOGY SERIES

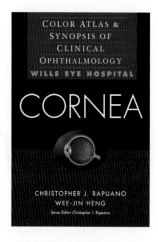

CORNEA
Christopher J. Rapuano, MD
Wee-Jin Heng, MD
0-07-137589-9

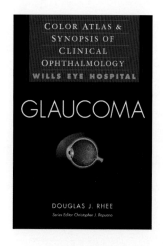

GLAUCOMA
Douglas J. Rhee, MD
0-07-137597-X

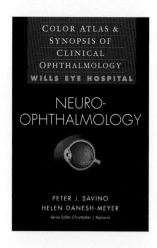

NEUROOPHTHALMOLOGY
Peter J. Savino, MD
Helen Danesh-Meyer, MD
0-07-137595-3

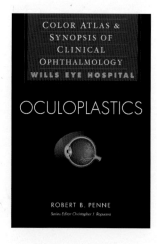

OCULOPLASTICS
Robert B. Penne, MD
0-07-137594-5

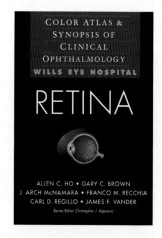

RETINA
Allen C. Ho, MD
Gary C. Brown, MD
J. Arch McNamara, MD
Franco M. Recchia, MD
Carl D. Regillo, MD
James F. Vander, MD
0-07-137596-1

COLOR ATLAS &
SYNOPSIS OF
CLINICAL
OPHTHALMOLOGY

WILLS EYE HOSPITAL

NEURO-OPHTHALMOLOGY

Peter J. Savino, MD

Director, Neuroophthalmology Service
Wills Eye Hospital
Professor of Ophthalmology and Neurology
Thomas Jefferson University
Philadelphia, PA

Helen V. Danesh-Meyer, FRANZCO

Sir William and Lady Stevenson Associate Professor of Ophthalmology,
Department of Ophthalmology
University of Auckland, New Zealand

McGraw-Hill
MEDICAL PUBLISHING DIVISION

New York   Chicago   San Francisco   Lisbon   London
Madrid   Mexico City   Milan   New Delhi   San Juan
Seoul   Singapore   Sydney   Toronto

Neuroophthalmology: Color Atlas and Synopsis of Clinical Ophthalmology

34567890   IMA/IMA   0987

ISBN 0-07-137595-3

This book was set in Times Roman by NK Graphics.
Prepress work was done by Accu-Color.
The editors were Darlene Cooke, Susan Noujaim, and Regina Brown.
The production supervisor was Philip Galea.
The book designer was Marsha Cohen.
The cover designer was Mary Belibasakis.
The index was prepared by Robert Swanson.
Imago, Singapore, was the printer and binder.

This book is printed on acid-free paper.

NOTICE

LIBRARY OF CONGRESS CATALOGING-IN-PUBLICATION DATA

Savino, Peter J.
    Color atlas and synopsis of clinical neuro-opthalmology / Peter J. Savino, Helen Danesch-Meyer.
      p.   cm.
    Includes bibliographical references and index.
    ISBN 0-07-137595-3 (softcover)
      1. Neuroophthalmology.   Neuroophthalmology—Atlases.   I. Danesh-Meyer, Helen.
    II. Title
      [DNLM: 1. Eye Diseases—Atlases. 2. Eye Manifestations—Atlases. 3. Nervous System Diseases—complications—Atlases. 4. Neurologic Manifestations—Atlases. 5. Optic Nerve Diseases—Atlases. WW 17 S267c 2003]
    RE725.S28 2003
    617.7—dc21

                                  2002069646

DEDICATION

To Marie and Mike
Juliette and Emily

CONTENTS

CONTRIBUTORS

Jurij R. Bilyk, MD

Assistant Professor of Ophthalmology
Thomas Jefferson University School of Medicine
Philadelphia, Pennsylvania
(Chapters 5 and 13)

Adam E. Flanders, MD

Professor of Radiology
Thomas Jefferson University School of Medicine
Philadelphia, Pennsylvania
(Chapter 3)

Jeffrey L. Friedman, MD

Fellow in Radiology
Thomas Jefferson University School of Medicine
Philadelphia, Pennsylvania
(Chapter 3)

Jean K. Yi, MD

Assistant Professor of Radiology
Thomas Jefferson University School of Medicine
Philadelphia, Pennsylvania
(Chapter 3)

ABOUT THE SERIES

The beauty of the atlas/synopsis concept is the powerful combination of illustrative photographs and a summary approach to the text. Ophthalmology is a very visual discipline which lends itself nicely to clinical photographs. While the five ophthalmic subspecialties in this series, Cornea, Retina, Glaucoma, Oculoplastics, and Neuroophthalmology employ varying levels of visual recognition, a relatively standard format for the text was used for all volumes.

The goal of the series is to provide an up-to-date clinical overview of the major areas of ophthalmology for students, residents, and practitioners in all the healthcare professions. The abundance of large, excellent quality photographs and concise, outline-form text will help achieve that objective.

Christopher J. Rapuano, MD
Series Editor

PREFACE

We undertook the task of writing this atlas to be part of a larger work, that of the Wills Eye Hospital Multi-Specialty Atlas series. Being part of a larger work and the format in which it was produced, required that we deal with certain limitations.

The book is an atlas, and therefore, cannot be encyclopedic so that certain information had to be omitted. We chose to include those topics that are the most frequently encountered entities in neuro-ophthalmology. These are problems that can face the general ophthalmologist on any given day in the office. We have tried to include the most clinically relevant material in each topic. We have purposely omitted the more exotic neuro-ophthalmologic syndromes.

Because the atlas series is a smaller soft-covered publication designed to be portable, certain limitations were imposed on the photographic array. We could not present some of the multiple series of eye movement disorders in more standard ways, but hope that the way we have displayed them makes sense to the reader and is not confusing or obfuscating.

Some of the photos may be smaller than we would ideally like, but in order to have a full exposition of the photographic variations of an entity (ocular motility, visual field, and neuroimaging) we chose to make them smaller and try to include them in one area, ideally on one page, so the reader would not be constantly flipping back and forth between text and photographs.

We hope that our compromises to the format have not sacrificed clarity and ease of reading and interpretation.

We include two invited chapters, one on basic MRI information for the general ophthalmologist, kindly written by Drs. Adam E. Flanders, Jeffrey L. Friedman, and Jean K. Yi from the Division of Neuro-Radiology at Thomas Jefferson University.

A chapter on orbital disorders with neuroophthalmologic implications is authored by Jurij R. Bilyk, M.D. of the Oculoplastic Service at Wills Eye Hospital. He also authored the section on Traumatic Optic Neuropathy in Chapter 5.

We express our gratitude to these authors for their willingness to contribute to the atlas, and to their flexibility in tailoring their chapters to our format.

This atlas could not have come to completion without the involvement of Jack Scully of the Audio-Visual Department at Wills Eye Hospital. His expertise, tireless dedication to making the photographs in this atlas as good as they could be, and his incredible good humor over many months in dealing with the authors is greatly appreciated. He literally had a role in the exposition of every single photograph in this atlas.

We hope that the work will be useful to residents in ophthalmology, and will be helpful to the practicing ophthalmologist. If we have accomplished this, we have succeeded in our task.

Peter J. Savino, M.D.
Helen Danesh-Meyer, FRANZCO

COLOR ATLAS &
SYNOPSIS OF
CLINICAL
OPHTHALMOLOGY

WILLS EYE HOSPITAL

NEURO-
OPHTHALMOLOGY

Chapter 1

EXAMINATION OF THE AFFERENT VISUAL SYSTEM

The purpose of the neuroophthalmic examination is to detect visual abnormalities (acuity or visual field) and to determine if they are due to neuroophthalmic disorders. The neuroophthalmic examination should be preceded by a thorough history of the presenting complaint, a detailed past medical history, social history, ocular history, list of medications, and review of systems. These procedures should be followed by a comprehensive ophthalmologic assessment that may identify non-neuroophthalmic causes for the visual disturbance (eg, microhyphema as a cause of transient visual loss). Only the parts of the examination that are directly relevant to the neuroophthalmic examination will be discussed in this chapter.

3. Bright light near vision. An improved near acuity with appropriate reading glasses and a bright light indicates the cause of decreased vision is refractive or cataractous.

4. Potential acuity devices: a variety of apparati project images (Snellen optotypes or lines) directly on the retina, thus, bypassing any refractive or media cause for decreased vision.

Improvement in visual acuity with any of these methods obviates the need to search for a neuroophthalmic cause of visual loss. Failure to improve the acuity, on the other hand, means further investigations for other causes, including neuroophthalmic diseases, are in order.

Visual Acuity

Patients can have decreased acuity from a variety of causes. The starting point of the neuroophthalmologic examination is to determine the *best-corrected* Snellen acuity. A variety of targets can be used to test visual acuity at distance (Figure 1–1). Several methods may be used to determine if the visual acuity can be improved and what is the likely cause of the poor vision.

1. Refraction
2. Pinhole: a series of pinholes measuring 2 to 2.5 mm are placed before each eye as its fellow is occluded (Figure 1–2). Improvement in acuity with pinhole indicates a refractive or media (eg, cataract) cause of decreased vision.

Color Vision

The purpose of color vision testing is to detect acquired unilateral or bilateral color loss, which occurs with optic neuropathies, disorders of the optic chiasm, and, more infrequently, with some occipital disorders (see Chapter 7). Most optic neuropathies produce marked loss of color perception; whereas in retinal or macular disease, the acuity may be poor but color vision is relatively preserved. Acquired dyschromatopsia is a useful clinical finding to support the presence of an optic nerve disorder.

Color vision may be tested with:

1. Ishihara pseudo-isochromatic plates: the patient is asked to identify the numbers displayed using each eye in turn (Figure 1–3).

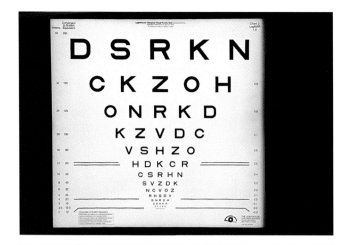

Figure 1–1. *The retro-illuminated Bailey–Lovie chart is placed at a distance of 4 m from the patient.*

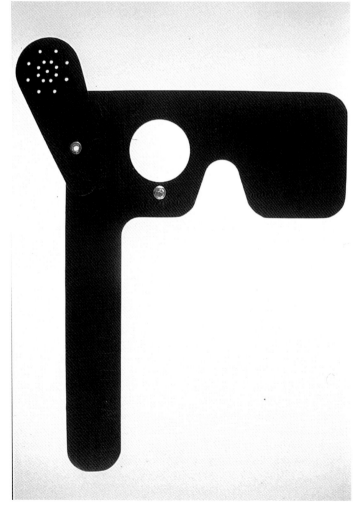

Figure 1–2. *Occluder with pin-holes that can be rotated into position in lieu of performing a refraction.*

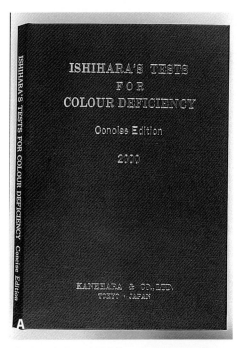
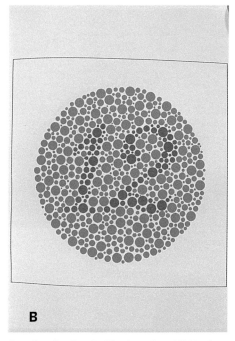

Figure 1–3. *A. Ishihara's pseudoisochromatic color-plate book.* ***B.*** *The first plate (12) is the control plate and is recognizable except with profound visual loss.*

This tests predominantly red-green color deficiencies.

2. Farnsworth panel D15: This panel has 15 caps with colors that are to be placed in order, starting with the closest hue to the reference cap, until all 15 are placed in sequence. A number on the back of each cap indicates its correct position in a normal sequence. This test identifies tritan (blue), deutan (green), and protan (red) color anomalies.

3. Farnsworth Munsel 100 hue: This tests actually consists of 85 (not 100) caps in four boxes (Figure 1–4) and is similar in concept to the D15 test. The 100-hue test can determine the severity as well as the axis of color anomaly. The FM 100 most thoroughly assesses color vision, but because it is tedious and cumbersome, it is not usually performed as a first-line color vision test.

4. Color comparison: at times, asking the patient to determine the amount of red in a test object (mydriatic bottle cap) with each eye to detect the percentage of red desaturation (eg, OD 100% OS 75%) will reveal subtle color anomalies (Figure 1–5). This is a highly subjective test, however, and further, more objective documentation of a color anomaly is preferable.

Pupillary Testing

Testing for the presence of a relative afferent pupillary defect (RAPD) should be performed on every patient. A bright light, either a halogen muscle light or indirect ophthalmoscope, is shone in each eye separately. The light illuminates each eye for the same amount of time (prolonged illumination of one eye may bleach the retina asymmetrically and produce a RAPD when none exists) and is swung between the eyes rapidly. Normal pupils will not dilate or constrict after the initial illumination under these circumstances. Unilateral decreased afferent input to the midbrain pupillomotor centers

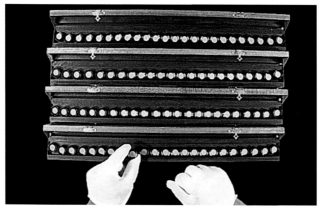

Figure 1–4. *The patient uses gloves and under standard illumination is asked to arrange the caps in sequence with respect to the color reference cap in each box.*

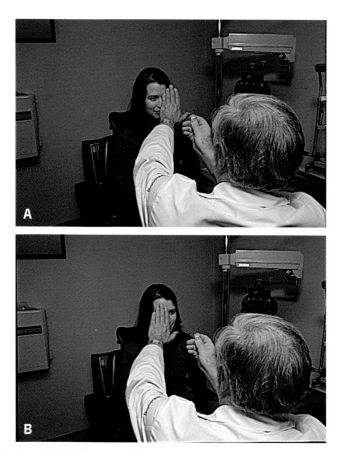

Figure 1–5. *A. and B. Color comparison.*

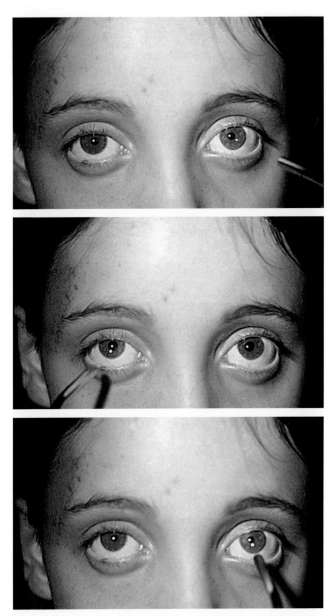

Figure 1–6. *Both pupils constrict when the light is directed into the left eye, but they both dilate when it is swung to the right eye. Both constrict again when the light is swung back to the left eye.*

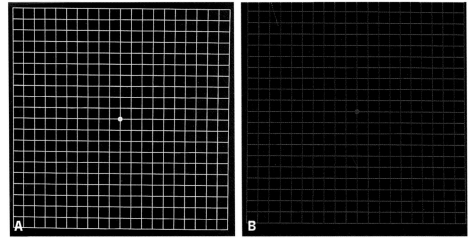

Figure 1–7. *A series of test plates can be used but the red and white squares on a black background are most useful.*

will produce a weaker pupillary contraction on the affected side. When the light swings to the normal pupil, both pupils constrict. Swinging back to the affected side causes both pupils to dilate (Figure 1–6).

The RAPD may be produced by:

1. Anterior chamber or vitreous hemorrhages
2. Large retinal detachments or macular lesions
3. Optic nerve disorders
4. Chiasmal compromise   RAO
5. Optic tract lesions

The RAPD is not produced by:

1. Cataract
2. Refractive errors
3. Lesions posterior to the lateral geniculate body
4. Nonphysiologic visual loss

Amsler Grid

The Amsler grid consists of a central dot for fixation surrounded by squares. The patient is instructed to look only at the central dot and to report (or draw) any scotomas or other alterations of the grid. Defects may be due to neuroophthalmic or retinal disease. The presence of metamorphopsia is an indication of a retinal and not an optic nerve abnormality. We find it useful to use the red grid on the black page as the first test since patients with subtle optic neuropathies may have a normal white on black Amsler but an abnormal red on black Amsler (Figure 1–7). If the red Amsler is normal, the white need not be tested.

The Amsler grid falls on the central area and encompasses 10 degrees around the fixation point. The optic disc, and thus the blind spot, is 5 degrees outside the temporal border of the grid.

Contrast Sensitivity (Figure 1–8)

Snellen acuity is routinely tested in a high-contrast setting (black letters on a white background). Decreasing the contrast can expose visual defects that may otherwise go undetected. Patients with optic neuritis, for example, often have poor contrast sensitivity despite "normal" acuity and color vision. A variety of methods may be used to test contrast sensitivity. We do not test it on all patients but find it useful in patients with visual complaints but with an otherwise normal examination.

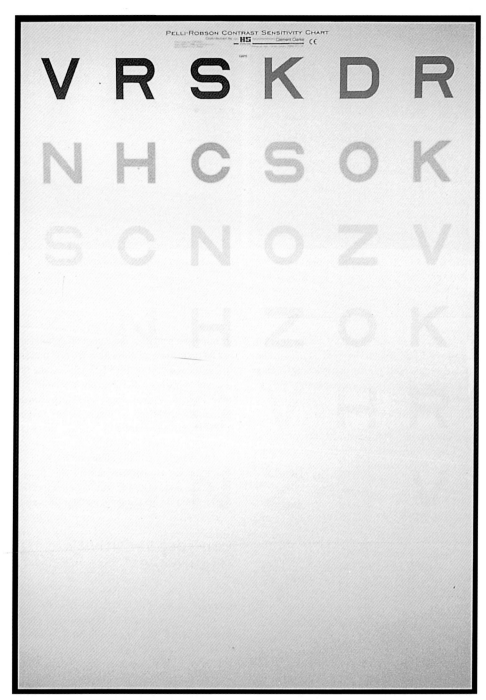

Figure 1–8. *The Pelli–Robson chart consists of 16 triplets of letters that gradually decrease in contrast. A normal response is correctly identifying 14 of the 16 triplets.*

Brightness Comparison

A simple comparison of brightness sensitivity between the two eyes is a sensitive test of a unilateral optic neuropathy. A light (from a muscle light or indirect ophthalmoscope) is shone directly into each eye separately. Care must be taken to shine the light directly along the visual axis in both eyes as shining the light obliquely in one eye will influence the patient's response. The patient is then asked the following questions: (1) Is the light equal between the two eyes or is one brighter? If one is brighter, then the patient is asked (2): If you give the value of 100 to the brighter light, what value would you give to the light when it is shone in the other eye? Alternatively, "If the light in the brighter eye is worth one dollar, how much is the light in the other eye worth?"

If the answer to question 1 was that the light in both eyes is equal, this makes an optic neuropathy as the cause for the visual disturbance less likely.

Photostress Recovery Test

This is a useful test to help differentiate between retinal disease and an optic neuropathy. The principle underlying this test is that recovery of retinal sensitivity following exposure to a bright light is based on regeneration of visual pigments that were bleached during the exposure to light. A delay in this process occurs in diseases that affect the photoreceptors or the adjacent retinal pigment epithelium. It is independent of the neural pathway. The test is performed as follows on each eye independently.

1. Determine best corrected visual acuity (VA) in each eye.
2. Patient looks directly into bright light source held at 2 to 3 cm for 10 seconds.
3. Record the time taken for the return of VA to within one line of the best corrected acuity.

Most normal patients will have a recovery time of less than 30 seconds and the recovery time between eyes is within 10 seconds. Macular disease, but not optic nerve disease, may cause a prolongation in the photostress recovery time. This is particularly useful for unilateral or subtle macular diseases.

Ophthalmoscopy

Examination of the fundus is an essential part of the neuroophthalmic examination. This can be performed with direct or indirect ophthalmoscopy. We recommend assessment of the optic disc with a 60, 78, or 90-diopter hand-held lens that allows stereoscopic examination.

Other aspects of the neuroophthalmic examination are covered in other portions of the text.

- Visual fields (Chapter 2)
- Ocular motility (Chapter 7)

Chapter 2

VISUAL FIELDS

Testing visual fields is an integral part of the neuroophthalmologic examination in any patient with an afferent system problem. In fact, any patient who has decreased vision that cannot be explained on an ocular or refractive basis should have a visual field as the very next test.

Several aspects of the principles that contribute to visual field interpretation are:

1. *Extent* of the normal monocular visual field

   Nasally 60 degrees
   Superiorly 60 degrees
   Inferiorly 70 to 75 degrees
   Temporally 100 to 110 degrees

2. Retinal nerve fiber *anatomy*. The basis of visual field defects is the anatomic structure of the retinal nerve fibers. There are four groupings of retinal nerve fibers that enter the optic disc.

   a. The inferior retinal nerve fibers subserve the superior visual field.
   b. The superior retinal nerve fibers subserve the inferior visual field.
   c. Fibers coursing between the macula and the optic disc (the papillomacular bundle) subserve central vision.
   d. The nasal fibers enter the optic disc directly in a wedge-shaped pattern.

   The superior and inferior nerve fibers are formed into arcuate bundles that course around the papillomacular bundle to enter the optic nerve at the 12 and 6 o'clock positions. Peripherally in the retina, they join at a structure called the horizontal raphé. Fibers do not cross this raphé.

   Thus, lesions in the retina will produce the following visual field defects.

   a. Involvement of the arcuate nerve fiber bundles produces an arcuate visual field defect. The nasal most extent of a superior or inferior arcuate defect is the horizontal meridian (Figure 2–1).
   b. Involvement of the papillomacular bundle produces a central (Figure 2–2A) or a cecocentral (Figure 2–2B) scotoma.
   c. Involvement of the nasal wedge fibers produces a temporal wedge defect.

   Lesions of the optic disc will produce visual field defects identical to those of the retina. As the retinal fibers extend posteriorly through the optic nerve toward the chiasm, they rotate 90 degrees, and the macular fibers come to occupy the central core of the optic nerve. Therefore, lesions in the retrobulbar prechiasmal optic nerve tend to produce more central scotomas, while lesions of the intracranial prechiasmal optic nerve may even present a visual field defect that begins to respect the vertical meridian (see Chapter 5).

3. *Testing strategies.* A variety of testing strategies are available to explore the extent of the visual field. The specific technology used is less important than the goal that the method employed arrives at the correct answer as to the form and extent of any scotoma.

   The types of visual field examinations performed routinely in neuroophthalmologic practice are as follows:

   a. Confrontation Visual Fields We believe that confrontation fields should be performed on all patients even those without afferent complaints. The test is quickly performed and easily understood by most patients. It will identify gross scotomas, but with experience,

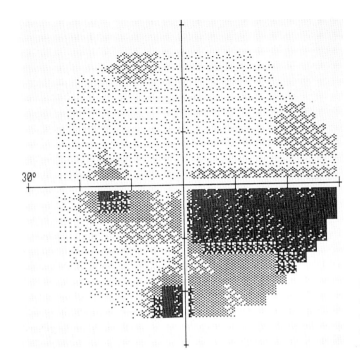

Figure 2-1. *A left inferior arcuate field defect denser nasally and respects the horizonal raphé.*

even smaller, more subtle scotomas may be identified.

The following technique to perform confrontation visual fields is recommended (Figure 2–3).

1. Examiner and patient are seated face to face at a distance of approximately 2 to 3 feet.
2. The patient is asked to occlude one eye using either the palm of his or her hand, a patch or other occluding device.
3. The patient is asked to fixate on the examiner's opposite eye (if patient's right eye is being examined, the patient fixates at the examiner's left eye) or nose.
4. A variety of targets can be employed. We use finger counting in the four quadrants,

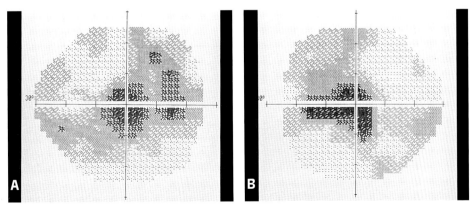

Figure 2-2. *A. Central scotoma right eye. The physiologic blind spot is separate from the scotoma.* *B. Cecocentral scotoma left eye involves the area of fixation and the physiologic blind spot.*

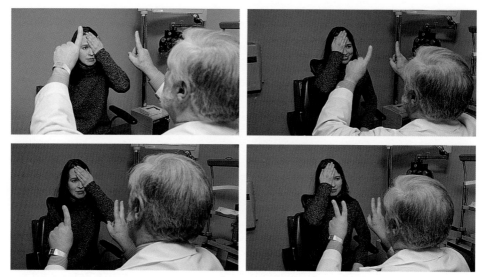

Figure 2–3. *Finger counting confrontation visual fields.*

testing across the horizontal midline and the vertical meridian. The examiner's fingers are presented in a plane halfway between the patient and examiner in all four quadrants. The patient is asked to indicate how many fingers are seen.

5. Simultaneous presentation of fingers in two quadrants can be used to speed up testing.

6. Patients needs to be told:
   a. This is a test of your side vision.
   b. Maintain central fixation (ie, look at examiner's eye) at all times and do not look at examiner's hands.

7. A red target, such as the top of a mydriatics bottle, is often used to test optic nerve function. Again, we present the red target in the four quadrants. Simultaneous comparison of color between hemifields and asking specifically about desaturation is useful in distinguishing subtle anomalies.

8. A modified version of the game, "Simon says" can be used for young children who cannot yet count fingers. The child is asked to mimic the examiner by holding up the same number of fingers as she observes (Figure 2–4).

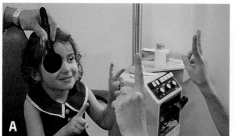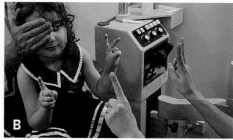

Figure 2–4. *A. The parent covers one eye as the child is asked to "do this" as fingers (usually 1, 2, or 5) are presented in the appropriate areas of visual field. **B.** If the child has difficulty fixing on the examiner's face, her head is turned so the eye is maximally abducted and she cannot move the eye laterally. This gives an accurate estimation of the temporal visual field.*

b. Static Automated Perimetry Automated perimetry has several advantages as a testing procedure. It is the most readily available means of visual field testing in most ophthalmology offices. It is not excessively technician-dependent, although some technician interaction during the testing procedure will ensure a more reliable result. It is a standardized method of testing and is an excellent way to follow visual fields to test for progression.

The most frequent testing strategy used is the thresholds strategy. Several sets of threshold strategies are available.

1. STATPAC: Conventional staircase strategy where threshold is crossed twice by changing the light in increments of 4 dB until the light is not seen and then increasing the light by 2 dB until it is seen again.
2. FASTPAC: Changes the intensity of the light by 3dB and only crosses the threshold once.
3. SITA (Swedish Interactive Threshold Algorithm): Uses a database of expected threshold values for patients with a more sophisticated knowledge of the relationship between different points and how they influence the outcome at other points. Hence, determination of the threshold is achieved by a few testing points.

Several programs are available on static threshold perimeters. We routinely employ three of them.

1. The full threshold 30-2, which consists of 76 testing points, and examines the full 30 degrees of visual field. The test points are spaced approximately 6-degrees apart.
2. The full threshold 24-2, which is similar to the 30-2 except that it eliminates the edge points, except for the two most nasal points along the horizontal meridian. Thus, 54 test points in the central 24 degrees are tested. The test points are likewise 6-degrees apart.
3. In order to magnify small, centrally located defects that might be missed on the 24-2 and the 30-2, the 10-2 program is used. This strategy tests all points within the 10 degrees of fixation in 2-degree intervals.

c. Kinetic Manual Perimetry (Goldmann Manual Perimetry) The perimeter designed by Goldmann is a bowl perimeter on which it is possible to perform both static and kinetic perimetry. The test can also explore the full extent of the visual field and is useful for testing for defects that occur outside the central 30-degree zone. The disadvantages of this technology are that it is becoming less available and is highly dependent on the skill of the perimetrist.

In this test, a super threshold object is moved from a peripheral area where the patient cannot perceive it toward the center of the visual field. The patient is instructed to signal as soon as the moving light is perceived. The speed at which the target moves is controlled by the examiner and must be constant.

d. Tangent Screen Many of the perimetric principles used today derive from testing with the tangent screen. This is a black felt covered board that measures the central 30 degrees of the visual field. The patient is seated in front of this large board while white or colored objects of specific sizes are brought in from the periphery to the center until the patient signals perception of the object. There are several disadvantages to this technique. The patient can tell from where the examiner is standing and where the examiner's arm is, the direction from whence the target is coming. In addition, the illumination is not standard. Finally, with loss of popularity of this method of testing visual fields, tangent screens are becoming less available.

With the tangent screen the distance that the patient sits from the testing surface can be changed. This is an important element in trying to detect nonphysiologic patterns of visual loss, such as tunnel vision.

Neuroophthalmologists tend to disagree about the types of visual fields that are best able to detect scotomas. Our bias is to perform 24-2 threshold tests as the mainstay of testing. If the patient is unable to perform that test, we utilize Goldmann perimetry if the patient can perform that test. In some patients, the only information that can be obtained about the visual field is by confrontation techniques.

Chapter 3

MAGNETIC RESONANCE IMAGING FOR THE OPHTHALMOLOGIST

The superior contrast resolution and multiplanar capabilities of magnetic resonance imaging (MRI) make it uniquely qualified for the assessment of the visual pathways. The predecessor to MRI, computed tomography (CT), also produces high-resolution digital images of the brain and orbital structures. However, because CT is based on the same physical principles of the x-ray, it accentuates bony anatomy at the expense of the soft-tissue detail. For example, at locations where soft tissue components of the orbital contents are in close approximation to bony elements (eg, the orbital apex, optic foramen) the details of the soft tissue structures are lost.

Mobile hydrogen protons generate images in MRI and these hydrogen protons are far more abundant in the soft tissue structures than in bone. Therefore, the soft tissues are accentuated in MRI at the expense of the bony anatomy. Thus, MRI is well suited for the detection of subtle abnormalities affecting the optic pathways. Disease processes that produce subtle pathologic changes in the optic pathways, such as optic neuritis, are easily identified with an MRI.

MRI uses a strong static magnetic field and radio waves to generate images; it has no known potential harmful effects in biologic tissues. Compared to CT, MRI does not use ionizing radiation; therefore, there is no potential risk of presenile cataracts due to radiation exposure for imaging the orbit. MRI does impose several safety limitations, which preclude imaging of patients with certain implanted ferrous instrumentation, such as cardiac pacemakers, neurostimulators, and older model cerebral aneurysm clips. In addition, approximately 10% of patients will experience an episode of claustrophobia during an MRI that may prevent completion of the entire examination. Sedation may be necessary in order to complete the examination.

High-field MRI units (one Tesla or greater) using a standard head (brain) coil can produce images of the optic pathways with exceptional detail. No special equipment is required. Although low-field strength open MRI units have become increasingly popular in recent years, their capabilities in resolving small structures (e.g., optic nerves, cranial nerves) is limited because of their low inherent magnetic field strength, longer imaging times, and lower spatial and contrast resolution. Use of these devices for ophthalmologic imaging should be reserved only as a last resort in preference to a high-field strength unit.

Fundamentals of Magnetic Resonance Imaging

MRI is based on the principles of nuclear magnetic resonance spectroscopy that have been in use by physical chemists for many years to deduce the chemical structure of unknown compounds; NMR, or nuclear magnetic resonance spectrometry. In brief, the images generated with MRI are created by exploiting the principle that the mobile protons in biologic tissues (primarily water and fat) align themselves and resonate along the direction of a strong static magnetic field at a known frequency (Larmour frequency). In a clinical MRI unit, the static magnetic field may vary between 0.3 to 3.0 Tesla (3000 to 30000 gauss—or up to 100,000 times the earth's own magnetic field). During the MR examination, the resonating protons are exposed to a burst of radiofrequency energy that briefly excites them to a higher energy state. After excitation, the protons spontaneously undergo a process of relaxation and release weak radiofrequency energy, which is detected by a large antenna (coil) inside the bore of the MRI unit. Through a series of sophisticated mathematical computations, the radio frequency map emitted by the excited tissue is converted into a spatial signal map that appears as an image.

Terminology

In the MRI unit, different tissues and disease processes exhibit *tissue specific relaxation properties* that allow one tissue to be distinguished from another. These fundamental relaxation properties are expressed as a rate or units of time and are known as *T1* and *T2* (Figure 3–1). Tissues can be described by their T1 and T2 relaxation rates, proton density and rate of movement (diffusion or blood flow). MRI pulse sequences (MR experiments) are designed to make use of tissue specific characteristics (eg, T1, proton density, flow, T2, and so forth) that improve the conspicuity of particular tissue relative to the background tissues. There is a large lexicon of pulse sequences; each sequence is designed to take advantage of particular tissue characteristics that allow a specific type of tissue or disease process to appear more noticeable than the remainder of the tissues. Many of the pulse sequences are specific to a given manufacturer and are identified by a confusing array of acronyms (such as SE, IR, RARE, FSE, FISP, FLASH, SMASH, SENSE, FLAIR, GRASS, SPGR, etc). A detailed discussion of these pulse sequences is beyond the scope of this chapter.

The basic pulse sequences take advantage of differences in the T1 or T2 relaxation properties, otherwise known as T1-weighted or T2-weighted pulse sequences. The term "weighted" is used because while the T1 or T2 relaxation characteristics provide the majority of the tissue information, there are other tissue-specific parameters that provide minor but observable contributions to the "look" of the images. It is useful to learn how to recognize these basic image types.

One of the most essential image types is the *T1 weighted image (T1WI)*. Characteristic of this type of image is that fat exhibits the highest signal intensity (bright) and the water containing structures (eg, the ventricles, the vitreous) exhibit low-signal intensity (dark). The myelinated white matter tracts that have higher intrinsic lipid content have slightly increased signal intensity than the gray matter. The T1WI is an essential part to any MR examination because it provides detailed normal and abnormal anatomic information see Figure 3–1A, B), (Figure 3–2A, B). Additionally, the T1-weighted image is used in conjunction with the MRI contrast agent, gadolinium, to identify and differentiate normal (see Figure 3–1 F–J) from abnormal pathologic enhancement.

In comparison to the T1WI, the *T2 weighted image (T2WI)* emphasizes structures, which contain abundant water. In this type of image, water-containing structures generally exhibit the highest signal intensity and the fat-containing structures yield relatively low-signal intensity. Since the white matter tracts contain relatively higher concentrations of lipid, they have relatively diminished signal intensity compared to gray matter on T2WI (see Figure 3–1C, D, E). In general, most pathologic processes have an increase in water content compared to normal tissues. For example, demyelinating lesions associated with optic neuritis and multiple sclerosis are secondary to the breakdown of normal myelin. Therefore, the demyelinating lesions have slightly increased water content relative to normal white matter which results in their characteristic abnormal high signal intensity on T2WI (Figure 3–3A). This property is also true for tumors (Figure 3–4D; 3–5A) and strokes (Figure 3–6A).

Intravenous contrast material is used to improve the visibility of an abnormality (eg, perioptic meningioma; Figure 3–7A–D; 3–8A, B),

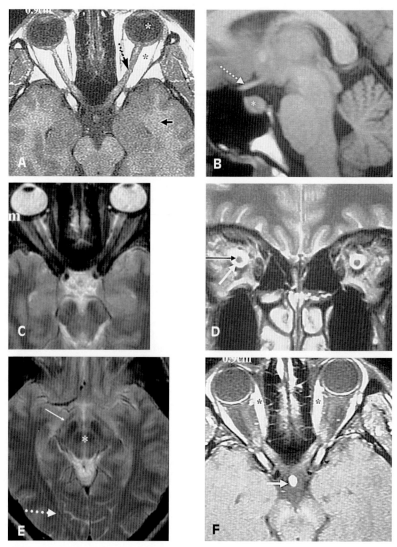

Figure 3–1. *A. Normal anatomy. Axial T1-weighted image (T1WI). The vitreous body is low in signal (white∗). The orbital fat is hyperintense (black∗). The optic nerve is seen throughout its entire course* (dotted arrow). *The white matter is slightly hyperintense relative to gray matter* (short black arrow). ***B.*** *midline sagittal T1WI shows the optic tract* (dotted arrow) *coursing through the suprasellar cistern. Normal pituitary (∗).* ***C.*** *Comparable axial T2-weighted image (T2-WI) shows the hyperintense (bright) vitreous body. The orbital fat is low in signal as is the cerebral white matter.* ***D.*** *Coronal T2WI through the mid-orbit shows the hyperintense cerebrospinal fluid contained by the optic sheath* (white arrow) *surrounding the lower signal intensity optic nerve* (black arrow). *E. Axial T2WI at midbrain level shows the optic tracts* (white arrow). *Midbrain (*). Optic radiations in occipital pole* (dotted arrow). *F. Contrast enhanced axial T1-weighted image using fat suppression (T1WI +C FS). Note that the signal from orbital fat is suppressed (low signal). The extraocular musculature normally enhances (∗), while the optic nerve does not. The normal infundibular enhancement* (white arrow).

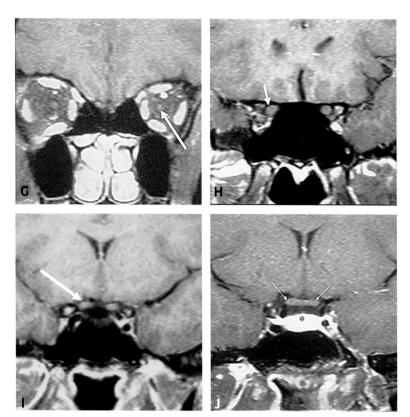

Figure 3–1. (*continued*) *G. Coronal T1WI +C FS. Note lack of enhancement of optic nerve/ sheath complex* (white arrow). *H. Coronal T1WI +C FS image at the level of the orbital apex shows the intracanalicular segment of the optic nerve* (white arrow). *I. Coronal T1WI +C FS image at the level of the orbital apex shows the prechiasmal segment of the optic nerve* (arrow). *J. Coronal T1WI +C FS image at the level of the optic chiasm* (arrows). *Note the normal enhancing pituitary gland* (*).

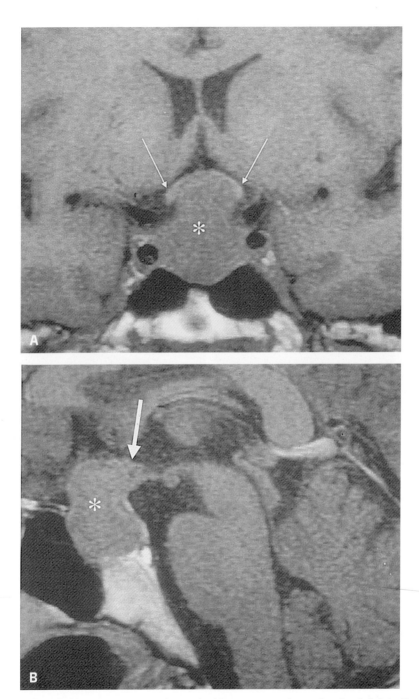

Figure 3-2.   *A. Pituitary tumor causing optic chiasm compression and a visual deficit. Coronal T1WI shows a bilobed, low-signal intensity mass (∗) that originates from the sella and extends superiorly. Note the compression of the optic nerves* (arrows).   *B. Sagittal T1WI shows the elevation of the optic apparatus* (arrow) *by the pituitary tumor.*

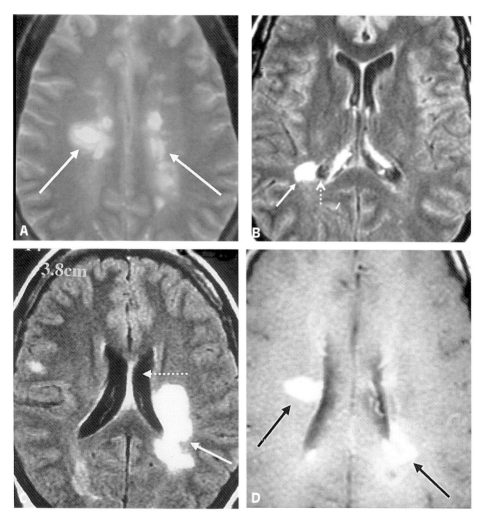

Figure 3–3. *A. Multiple sclerosis. Axial T2WI at the level of centrum semiovale demonstrates multiple, round periventricular white matter high-signal intensity lesions consistent with demyelinating plaques* (arrows). *B. Axial FLAIR image demonstrates a periventricular white matter high-signal intensity lesion* (arrow) *consistent with a demyelination plaque. Note the attenuation of the cerbrospinal fluid signal* (vertical arrow) *compared to the T2WI in A. C. Axial FLAIR image in another patient demonstrates a large periventricular white matter high-signal intensity lesion* (solid arrow) *consistent with tumefactive demyelination related to multiple sclerosis. Note the cerebrospinal fluid signal attenuation* (dotted arrow). *D. Axial T1WI +C in another patient shows enhancing multiple sclerosis plaques* (arrows)

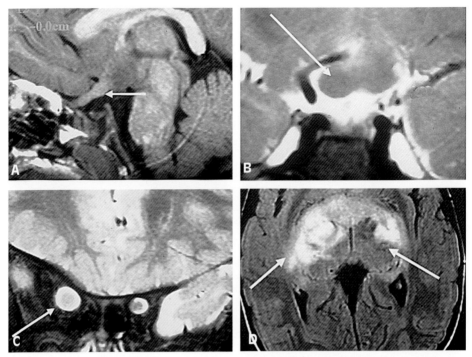

Figure 3-4. *A. Optic glioma in neurofibromatosis type I. Sagittal T1WI shows enlargement of the optic chiasm and tract (arrow).* ***B.*** *Coronal T2WI shows the bulbous optic chiasm and nerves (arrow).* ***C.*** *Coronal T2WI of the optic canal shows the dilated optic nerve sheath and enlarged optic nerve (arrow).* ***D.*** *Axial FLAIR image at the level of the basal ganglia show the characteristic hamartomas of the base of the brain and optic tracts (arrows).*

to characterize the activity of a pathologic process [eg, multiple sclerosis (Figure 3–3D), or to make pathology visible (eg, optic neuritis (Figure 3–9A–D)]. With the possible exception of imaging for optic atrophy, use of contrast material is mandatory when imaging the optic pathways. The mechanism for contrast enhancement in MRI is similar to the process on CT; it augments areas of increased vascularity or vascular permeability (eg, damaged blood–brain barrier). The active material in the MR contrast agent is the heavy metal gadolinium. When this agent escapes from the capillary bed into the interstitium either by a relative increased pathologic vascularity or by "leaky" capillary endothelium, it alters the T1 relaxation parameters of the local tissues in such a way that tissues containing minute quantities of the

agent will appear relatively hyperintense (brighter) than surrounding normal tissue. Since the physiologic basis for enhancement (ie, alteration in vascularity and capillary permeability) is present with a number of pathologic entities, the enhancement on contrast MRI is not specific for any particular disease process.

A fat suppression technique is mandatory in the evaluation of the orbit to augment the effects of the gadolinium contrast agent. Subtle areas of contrast enhancement can often be difficult to identify on a standard T1WI in the orbit because of the intense signal from the orbital fat. Therefore, it is often necessary to obtain images that actively suppress the dominant signal created by the orbital fat. Fat suppression can be performed in both T1- and T2-weighted images. Fat suppression in T1-weighted images is im-

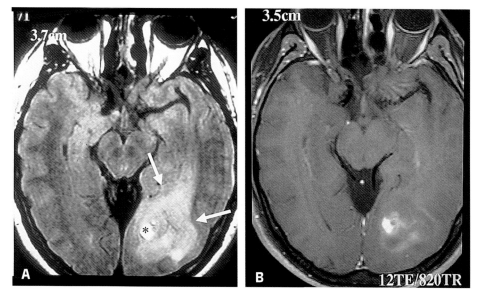

Figure 3–5. *A. Occipital lobe glioma producing a visual field cut. Axial FLAIR image of the brain reveals an infiltrative mass in the left occipital pole* (arrows) *with a small internal focus of hemorrhage (∗). **B.** Axial T1WI +C shows vague enhancement of the mass.*

portant in distinguishing fatty lesion from other lesions that have increased signal intensity on T1WI such as subacute hemorrhage. In general, the ability to perceive an abnormality is markedly improved with the use of a fat suppression technique. This option is standard on all high-field strength systems. The use of this technique is necessary when searching for intraorbital masses, optic neuritis (Figure 3–9A–D), and perioptic meningiomas (Figure 3–7A–D). The fat suppression in T2-weighted images is used to better delineate edema and excess water. The pathologic lesions usually have excess water content, thus, with T2-weighted fat-suppressed images, excess water can be better defined. Rules of MRI interpretation, therefore, are largely dependent on the location and morphology of the abnormality in conjunction with the clinical history (Figure 3–2A,B; 3–8A,B).

One particular pulse sequence acronym that has become ubiquitous is FLAIR, or fluid attenuated inversion recovery. This technique can be used to obtain either T1- or T2-weighted images, however, it is most commonly used to

obtain T2-weighted information. The FLAIR T2WI actively suppresses the signal arising from bulk water (cerebrospinal fluid) more than from bound water (interstitial edema or demyelination). This is the most sensitive technique to demonstrate periventricular white matter disease [eg, demyelinating lesions, ischemia (see Figure 3–3B,C; 3–6A)] and subarachnoid disease processes (eg, subarachnoid hemorrhage and leptomeningeal inflammation or carcinomatosis).

One of the most clinically useful pulse sequences is based on the physiologic process of molecular diffusion. The diffusion-weighted image (DWI) is founded on the principal that cytotoxic edema (from cellular swelling) produces slow diffusion of molecules into the cells due to intracellular water accumulation. This produces increased signal on the DWI images. This technique is the most sensitive method for the identification of acute cerebral cortical infarction (see Figure 3–6B). DWI can be abnormal within few minutes of the ictus. Moreover, a stroke may manifest itself on DWI without a

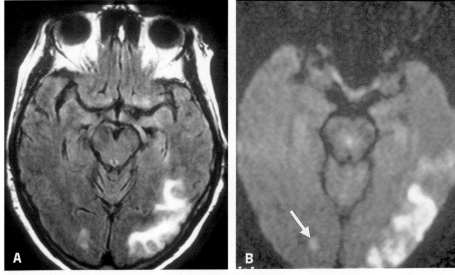

Figure 3–6. *A. Acute occipital infarction. Axial FLAIR image shows a large hyperintense region involving the cortex and subcortical white matter of the left occipital pole consistent with an infarction.* *B. Corresponding axial diffusion-weighted image shows an area of restricted diffusion that signifies the infarction is relatively recent. Note the smaller acute infarct in the right occipital pole* (arrow).

corresponding abnormality on the conventional MR images. The intensity of the signal decreases several days after the ictus and can persist up to 4 to 6 weeks. Although DWI is most useful in diagnosing strokes, it can be helpful in defining abscess, a number of active demyelinating plaques, and certain tumors.

Protons in motion exhibit a specific type of signature that can be exploited with MRI. The MR techniques that are used to image flowing blood are collectively known as magnetic resonance angiography (MRA). With this technique, the signal from fast-moving particles, such as blood, is augmented while the signal from the stationary tissues is suppressed. The images are acquired without intravenous contrast agent, and are post-processed to produce an angiographic-like image. This method has evolved to a level where it is now used to replace conventional catheter angiography in specific applications. This technique is a useful noninvasive procedure in diagnosing intracranial aneurysms (Figure 3–10A–C), strokes, ath-

erosclerotic disease, venous thrombosis (Figure 3–11A–C), and large vascular malformations.

Recommended Imaging Protocol

A suggested imaging protocol for use in imaging the optic pathways should include the following.

1. Sagittal T1 of entire brain by 5-mm slice thickness.
2. Axial T1- and T2-weighted images parallel to the optic nerves by 3-mm slice thickness.
3. Coronal fast-spin echo T2- and T1-weighted image through the optic nerves up to the optic tracts by 3-mm slice thickness.
4. Axial FLAIR of the entire brain by 5-mm slice thickness.
5. Axial DWI of the entire brain by 5-mm slice thickness.
6. Intravenous gadolinium (0.1 mmol/kg).

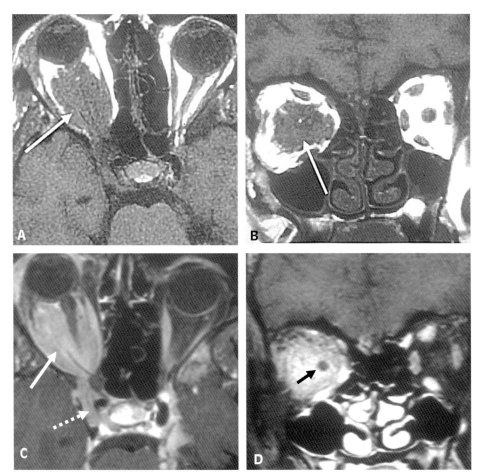

Figure 3–7. *A. Perioptic meningioma. Axial T1WI shows an irregularly shaped mass encasing the optic nerve (arrow). **B.** Coronal T1WI. **C.** Axial T1WI +C FS shows the marked enhancement of the mass (arrow) with extension through the optic canal into the cavernous sinus (dotted arrow). **D.** Coronal T1WI +C FS. Note the absence of enhancement of the optic nerve sheath compared to the mass (arrow).*

7. Post contrast fat-suppressed axial and coronal T1-weighted images through the optic nerve up to the optic tracts by 3-mm slice thickness.

8. Sagittal oblique T1-weighted images oriented parallel to the course of the optic nerve (optional).

9. Post contrast axial of the entire brain by 5-mm slice thickness.

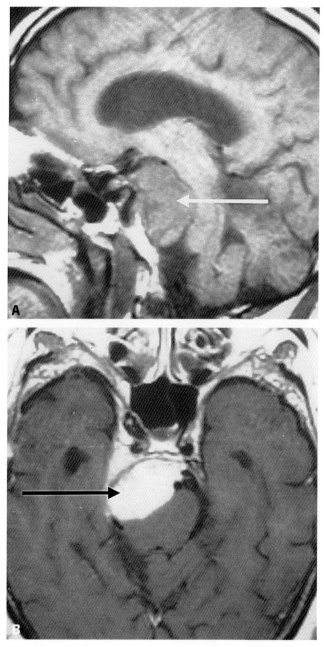

Figure 3–8. *A. Clivus meningioma producing a right abducens palsy. Sagittal T1WI shows a large mass* (arrow) *originating from the clivus extending into the prepontine cistern causing compression of the brainstem.* *B. Axial T1WI +C shows the characteristic intense enhancement of the meningioma.*

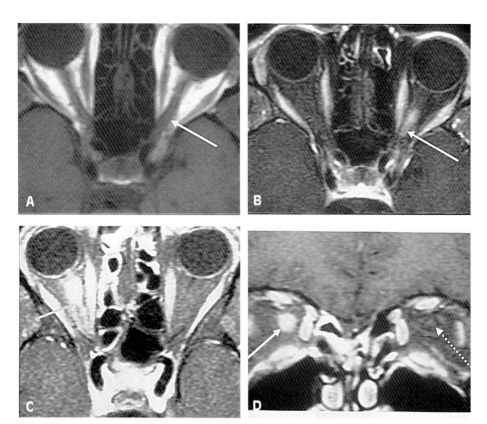

Figure 3–9.   *A–D. Optic neuritis.*   **A.** *Axial T1WI demonstrates a focally enlarged optic nerve* (arrow).   **B.** *Comparable, Axial T1WI + C FS, demonstrates abnormal left optic nerve enhancement* (arrow).   **C.** *Axial T1WI + C FS on another patient demonstrates an enlarged enhancing right optic nerve* (arrow) *consistent with optic neuritis.*   **D.** *Coronal T1WI + C FS demonstrates an enlarged enhancing optic nerve* (arrow) *consistent with optic neuritis; the left optic nerve* (dotted arrow) *does not enhance.*

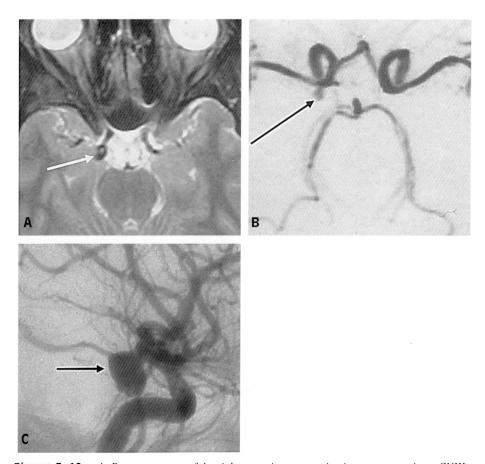

Figure 3–10. *A. Berry aneurysm of the right posterior communicating artery causing a CNIII palsy. Axial T2WI shows an oval shaped structure with no internal signal* (arrow) *projecting posteriorly from the right internal carotid artery.* *B. Magnetic resonance angiogram (axial projection) confirms that there is blood flow within the abnormality* (arrow). *C. Lateral projection from a conventional cerebral arteriogram shows filling of the posterior communicating artery aneurysm sac* (arrow).

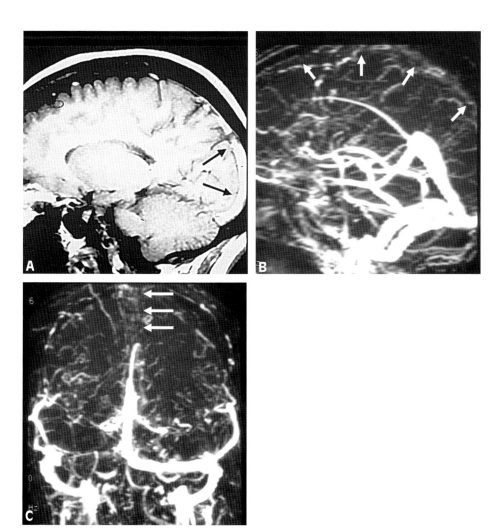

Figure 3–11. *Sagittal sinus thrombosis producing papilledema.* **A.** *Sagittal T1WI shows an arcuate shaped hyperintense band* (arrows) *representing thrombus in the sagittal sinus.* **B.** *Lateral view from MR venogram shows absence of signal in the expected location of the superior sagittal sinus* (arrows) *with normal definition of the other venous sinuses.* **C.** *Frontal view from MR venogram. Arrows indicate location of superior sagittal sinus. Flowing blood in normal veins appears white.*

Chapter 4

RETINAL ARTERY OCCLUSION

Occlusion of retinal arterioles in the form of a branch retinal artery occlusion (BRAO) or central retinal artery occlusion (CRAO) may be a precursor to further visual loss, stroke, or death.

Epidemiology and Etiology

The causes of retinal artery occlusion may be embolic or thrombotic. Different etiologies are more prevalent in different age groups. For example, in the vasculopathic age group (over 50 years of age), carotid atheroma is a more likely cause than it would be in a younger population. In the younger age group, hyperviscosity syndromes, vasculitis, or cardiac abnormalities tend to be more frequent causes.

Clinical Characteristics

Symptoms The primary symptom is painless visual loss, which is sudden, but may be stepwise and stuttering in onset. The visual loss may be partial, with a scotoma that may involve or spare fixation, or may be nearly total, with the preservation of a small island of peripheral vision. The presence of a cilioretinal artery will often determine the configuration of the scotoma, and at times, the level of visual acuity.

Signs

1. Decreased acuity if the macula area is involved.
2. Visual field defects that correspond to the area of retinal infarction (Figure 4–1).
3. Relative afferent pupillary defect is usually detected.

4. Area of retinal whitening that corresponds to the scotoma is seen acutely, but fades over days or weeks (Figure 4–1, 4–2).
5. Intravascular embolic or thrombotic material, at times characteristic of its site of origin, is sometimes identified on ophthalmoscopy (Figure 4–3).
6. Diabetic patients with carotid occlusions will have less diabetic retinopathy to the side of the occluded carotid artery (Figure 4–4).

Investigations

Investigation depends on the age of the patient and the presence or absence of visible embolic material in the retinal circulation (Table 4–1). The presence of visible emboli dictates that the primary investigations be aimed at finding the source of the emboli. The studies that should be performed are:

1. Determination of carotid patency (MRA or carotid Doppler). The presence of a refractile embolus in the retinal circulation (Hollenhorst plaque) is highly suggestive of a cholesterol embolus originating in a carotid atheroma (Figure 4–4).
2. In younger patients, carotid atheromas are less likely to be the cause of retinal artery occlusion, and the investigation should focus primarily on:
   • Cardiac evaluation including echocardiography and rhythm monitoring.
   • Investigation for hyperviscosity states, especially including testing for the presence of anticardiolipin and anti-phospholipid antibodies.
   • Testing for underlying vasculitis.

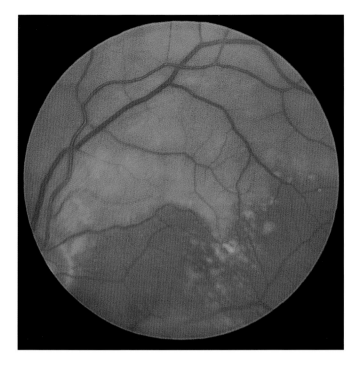

Figure 4–1. *Branch retinal artery occlusion with retinal whitening of the superior arcuate nerve fiber bundle. The patient had an inferior arcuate visual field defect.*

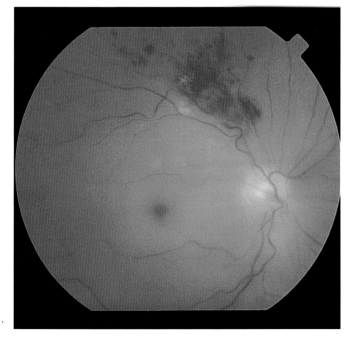

Figure 4–2. *Central retinal artery occlusion with a cherry red spot. Nerve fiber layer hemorrhages are seen superior to the disc.*

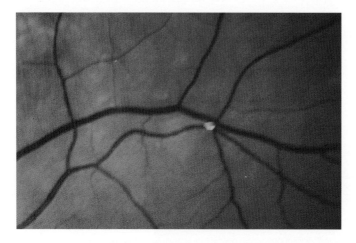

Figure 4–3. *A bright plaque that appears larger than the artery in which it resides is seen at a retinal arteriole bifurcation. This glistening appearance suggests a cholesterol embolus of carotid artery origin.*

3. In older patients without embolic material present in the retinal arterioles, giant cell arteritis (GCA) always must be considered, and the appropriate questions to detect this disorder should be asked. Any suspicion that GCA is the cause of the retinal artery occlusion, should prompt urgent treatment with systemic corticosteroids while temporal artery biopsy is performed (see p. 60).

Patients, especially diabetics, who have a retinal artery occlusion combined with ophthalmoplegia or other orbital signs, should be investigated for paranasal sinus fungal infection, for example, mucormycosis. Often the initial MRI or CT scan is normal or minimally abnormal.

Treatment

There is no unanimity of opinion on the usefulness of treatment of acute retinal artery occlusion. Traditional treatments include lowering the intraocular pressure to promote better intraocular perfusion. This is done by anterior chamber paracentesis or by administering pharmacologic agents that block aqueous secretion. Ocular massage is recommended on the assumption that it may dislodge an embolus and allow

TABLE 4–1   INVESTIGATION OF RETINAL ARTERY OCCLUSION

	Embolus Present	No Embolus Present
Under age 50	Cardiac echography Carotid Doppler/MRA	Cardiac echography Cardiac rhythm monitor Hyperviscosity panel
Over age 50	Carotid Doppler/MRA Cardiac echography	Cardiac echography Cardiac rhythm monitor Hyperviscosity panel Erythrocyte sedementation rate (ESR), Temporal Artery Biopsy (GCA)

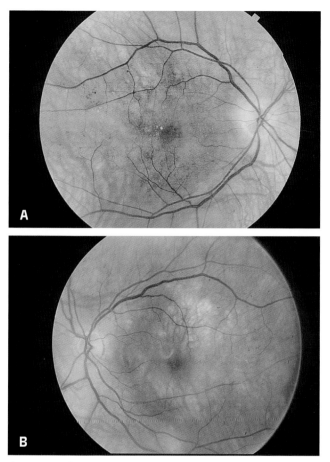

Figure 4–4. *A patient with diabetes has obvious diabetic retinopathy in the right eye (A), but none in the left (B). Because of this, carotid ultrasound was performed and carotid occlusion was documented on the left, but not on the right.*

reperfusion of the ischemic retina. Although no prospective studies prove that any of these maneuvers is helpful in restoring retinal blood flow, we believe that these maneuvers should be tried acutely, possibly up to 12 hours from the time of onset of the retinal artery occlusion.

Treatment varies depending on the underlying condition. There is controversy with regard to carotid stenosis. Prospective multicenter studies indicate that patients with carotid stenosis greater than 70% benefit more from surgical en-

darterectomy than from medical treatment. This presumes, however, a low rate of intra- and perioperative morbidity and mortality (under 2%). Surgical candidates should be in reasonably good health and have the anticipation of multiyear survival. Patients with visual transient ischemic attacks (TIA) may be at a lower risk for stroke than those with cerebral TIA. A more conservative therapeutic approach to patients with only visual symptoms may be indicated.

Chapter 5

OPTIC NERVE DISORDERS

OPTIC NEURITIS

The term optic neuritis most often refers to the optic neuropathy associated with demyelinating disease (multiple sclerosis (MS)). Demyelinating optic neuritis can be considered in three categories: acute, chronic or asymptomatic (subclinical). Acute optic neuritis is the most common form of optic neuritis.

Epidemiology and Etiology

1. Multiple sclerosis: optic neuritis may be the initial presentation of this disorder.
2. Age of onset: 20 to 50 years, mean age of 30 to 35 years.
3. Gender: more common in women.
4. Incidence: between 1 to 5 per 100,000.
5. Prevalence: approximately 115 per 100,000.

Clinical Characteristics

Symptoms

1. Pain or discomfort around the orbit or with eye movement is present in approximately 90% of patients. It may precede or occur concurrently with the visual loss.
2. Decreased acuity is the rule. The degree of visual loss varies widely and is usually monocular, although a small subgroup, particularly children, often have both eyes affected simultaneously.
3. Other: positive visual phenomena (photopsias), such as flashes of lights, showers of sparks or flashing black squares, may occur spontaneously or in response to loud noises.

Signs

1. A RAPD: if the process is unilateral or asymmetric.
2. Decreased visual acuity is the rule but need not be present.
3. Acquired dyschromatopsia with the color deficit often being greater than the degree of visual acuity loss.
4. Virtually any type of optic nerve visual field defect can occur in optic neuritis (Figure 5–1). Visual field defects are often found in the contralateral eye.
5. Contrast sensitivity impairment is found in virtually all patients with optic neuritis.
6. The optic disc appears normal (retrobulbar neuritis) in about two-thirds of patients. Optic disc swelling (Figure 5–2) will be present in 20 to 40% of cases. The degree of swelling does not correlate with the severity of optic nerve dysfunction. Optic disc or peripapillary hemorrhages are uncommon.

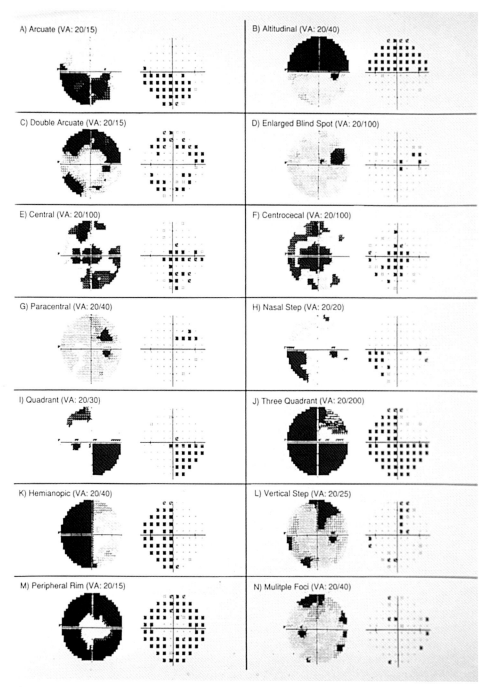

Figure 5–1. *Composite of visual field abnormalities found in the Optic Neuritis Treatment Trial (ONTT). (Keltner JL et al. Baseline Visual Field Profile of Optic Neuritis. Arch Ophthalmol 111:233, 1993 with permission).*

CHAPTER 5 OPTIC NERVE DISORDERS

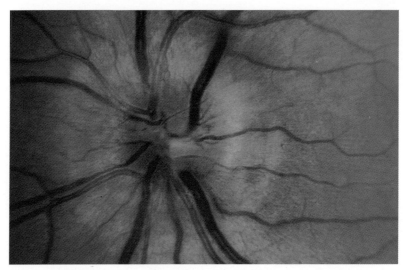

Figure 5–2. *The optic disc is elevated and hyperemic with opacification of the retinal nerve fiber layer. The fellow optic disc was normal.*

7. Vitreous cells, particularly overlying the optic disc, may be seen but are usually minimal.
8. Peripheral venous sheathing occurs in some patients with demyelinating optic neuritis.

Diagnosis and Investigations

1. Neuroimaging: MRI is the modality of choice for investigating optic neuritis. If the patient has a typical presentation of optic neuritis, an MRI need not be performed to exclude a compressive lesion or to confirm the diagnosis (which is made on clinical grounds). An MRI can be performed to detect subclinical demyelinating plaques (Figure 5–3) to:
   • Assist in determining the prognosis for developing MS.
   • Evaluate patient's potential benefit from intravenous methylprednisolone and intramuscular interferon beta-1a therapy.
2. Cerebrospinal fluid examination may be performed, however, this testing is not necessary and is being performed less frequently. The following abnormalities have been identified in patients with optic neuritis, although none is diagnostic of MS:
   • Pleocytosis and elevated protein
   • Oligoclonal bands
   • Myelin basic protein
   • Increased IgG index
3. Visual evoked responses (VER) are almost always abnormal, showing a prolonged latency on the side of the affected optic nerve.
4. No serologic tests or cerebrospinal fluid studies need to be performed unless the patient's course does not follow that of typical optic neuritis or the patient's history or examination suggests an underlying systemic illness (Table 5–1).

Treatment

1. There is no known treatment for optic neuritis. Fortunately, visual recovery is the rule, with approximately 90% of patients recovering to 20/40 or better vision within weeks.
2. Patients who have two or more periventricular white matter lesions are at an increased risk to develop MS. Administration of IV

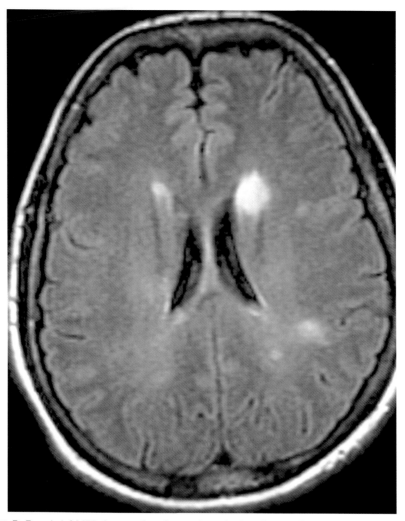

Figure 5–3. *Axial MRI shows enhancing periventricular plaques characteristic of MS.*

corticosteroids (1 g/day) for 3 days, followed by a 15-day schedule of oral prednisone and the institution of interferon beta-1a lowers the risk of developing MS over the next 3 years to 35%, instead of the 50% risk in untreated patients (see section, "Natural History of Optic Neuritis").

Natural History of Optic Neuritis

1. Initially, the visual loss may worsen over several days to 2 weeks.
2. Improvement initially is rapid and starts approximately 3 weeks after onset.
3. Recovery of vision is nearly complete by 5 weeks after onset.
4. Improvement continues up to 1 year.

TABLE 5–1. RESULTS OF INVESTIGATIONS OF PATIENTS IN OPTIC NEURITIS TREATMENT TRIAL

Etiologic studies
  ANA positive in titer <1:320 in 13%; one patient developed a connective tissue disorder within 2 years
  Chest radiograph: no case of sarcoidosis or TB was identified
  CSF analysis: no lumbar puncture offered any unsuspected information
  FTA-ABS: no case of active syphilis was identified

The present recommendations for the investigation and treatment of patients with optic neuritis are based on the results of two multi-centered studies, the ONTT and Controlled High Risk Subjects Avonex Multiple Sclerosis Prevention Study (CHAMPS). Both studies investigated the risk of developing clinically definite multiple sclerosis (CDMS) in patients with optic neuritis alone (ONTT) or with their first demyelinating episode that could be optic neuritis (CHAMPS). The details of the ONTT are listed in Table 5–2. The visual defects and their response to the treatment protocols are in Tables 5–3 and 5–4, respectively. The ONTT also calculated the risk of developing CDMS in patients with optic neuritis. The risk and the effect of treatment on these risks are shown in Table 5–5 and Figure 5–4. Table 5–6 shows the risk at the yearly follow-up periods.

The only accurate predictor of increased risk to develop CDMS was the number of lesions on the initial MRI scan (Figure 5–5.) The CHAMPS (Table 5–7) extended the ONTT by including other neurologic events (50% of the patients had optic neuritis) and investigated the efficacy of interferon beta-1a versus placebo both on the development of CDMS and on the development or evolution of MRI lesions (Figure 5–6). The results and conclusions of CHAMPS are listed in Tables 5–8 and 5–9.

TABLE 5–2. OPTIC NEURITIS TREATMENT TRIAL

Multicentered control clinical trial
 389 Patients with isolated acute unilateral optic neuritis between 18 and 46 years old
Inclusion criteria:
  Clinical syndrome consistent with unilateral optic neuritis (including RAPD, visual field defect in affected eye)
  Visual symptoms of 8 days or less
  No previous episode of optic neuritis in affected eye
  No previous corticosteroid treatment for optic neuritis or multiple sclerosis
  No evidence of systemic disease other than MS as a cause for optic neuritis.
Randomized to three treatment groups
  Oral prednisone 1 mg/kg per day for 14 days, plus short oral taper
  Intravenous methylprednisolone 250 mg QID for 3 days followed by 1 mg/kg per day for 11 days orally, plus a short taper
  Oral placebo for 14 days

TABLE 5–3. ONTT BASELINE DATA

Gender: 77% female
Race: 85% Caucasian
Age: mean 32±7 years
Symptoms:
  Photopsias 30%
  Orbital pain 92%
  Pain worsened with eye movement 87%
Signs:
  Baseline Visual acuity
    20/20 11%
    20/50–20/40 25%
    20/50–20/190 29%
    20/200–20/800 20%
    Finger counting 4%
    Hand motion 6%
    Light perception 3%
    No light perception 3%
  Color vision:
    Ishihara color plates abnormal 88%
    Farnsworth-Munsell 100 Hue abnormal 94%
  Visual Field
    Focal defects (altitudinal, arcuate, nasal step,
      central or paracentral defects) 52%
    Diffuse defects 48%
  Contrast sensitivity: abnormal 98%
Ophthalmoscopic appearance:
  Optic disc swelling 35%
  Optic disc or peripapillary hemorrhages 6%
Abnormal fellow eye:
  Visual activity 13.8%
  Contrast sensitivity 15.4%
  Color vision 21.7%
  Visual field 48%

TABLE 5–4. VISUAL RECOVERY

No significant difference between three arms of treatment groups at 1 year in mean VA, color vision, contrast sensitivity, or visual field

Patients treated with IV methylprednisolone recovered VA significantly faster than other two treatment arms; this affect was greatest in the first 15 days

Patients treated with oral prednisolone had an increased rate of recurrent attacks of optic neuritis in the previously affected eye and in the fellow eye

Median VA in all three treatment groups was 20/16

Less than 10% have VA 20/50 or worse

Of patients with baseline VA of worse than 20/200, 6% had this level of vision at 6 months

Of patient with initial VA of light perception or no light perception, 64% had a final VA of 20/40 or better

TABLE 5–5. CUMULATIVE RISK OF DEVELOPMENT OF MULTIPLE SCLEROSIS

Based on initial MRI results (at 4 years)
  13% with normal MRI
  35% with 1–2 lesions greater than 3 mm in size
  50% with more than 2 lesions greater than 3 mm in size
Based on treatment group
  Patients in the group treated with IV methylprednisolone had a reduced rate of development of MS
    during the first 2 years *only* in patients who had abnormal brain imaging at time of diagnosis
  The 2-year risk of MS was too low in patients with normal imaging to assess the value of treatment
  At 3 years, there was no significant difference in the rate of development of MS between the three
    treatment arms

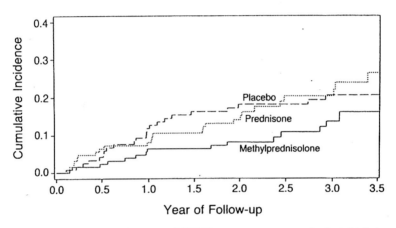

Figure 5–4. *Incidence of development of CDMS per treatment group in the initial phase of the ONTT. (Beck RW et al, NEJM 326:581–588, 1992 with permission).*

TABLE 5–6. CUMULATIVE PROBABILITY OF CLINICALLY DEFINITE MULTIPLE SCLEROSIS BY TREATMENT GROUP

Time Period	Treatment Group		
	Intravenous N = 133 (%)	Placebo N = 126 (%)	Oral Prednisone N = 129 (%)
6 mo	3.1	6.7	7.1
1 yr	6.4	12.6	10.4
2 yr	8.0	17.6	17.0
3 yr	18.5	21.0	24.5
4 yr	24.6	26.3	27.8
5 yr	26.4	31.1	32.1

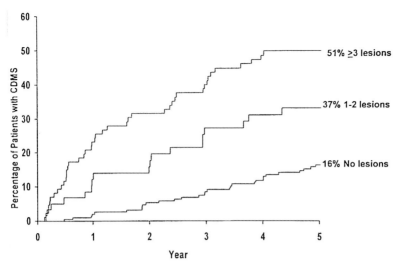

Figure 5–5. *Percentage of patients developing CDMS is directly related to the number of lesions on MRI. (The 5-year Risk of MS After Optic Neuritis. Neurology 49:1407, 1997 with permission).*

TABLE 5–7.   THE CHAMPS

Multicentered randomized double-blind control clinical trial
Eligibility criteria
  18 to 50 years old
  First isolated, well-defined neurologic event consistent with demyelination involving either: the optic nerve (optic neuritis), spinal cord (incomplete transverse myelitis), or brainstem or cerebellum
  MRI abnormality: two or more silent lesions of the brain at least 3 mm in diameter characteristic of MS
  Onset of symptoms 14 days or less before intravenous corticosteroid therapy and no more than 27 days before randomization
Treatment groups
  Interferon-beta-1a 30 μg weekly by intramuscular injection following intravenous methylprednisolone 1 g per day for 3 days with an 11-day subsequent oral prednisone 1 mg/kg
  Placebo intramuscular injection weekly following intravenous methylprednisolone 1 g per day for 3 days with an 11-day subsequent oral prednisone 1 mg/kg

TABLE 5–8. CHAMPS RESULTS

Cumulative probability of development of CDMS during the 3-year follow-up period was significantly lower in the interferon-beta-1a group (adjusted rate ratio, 0.49; 95% CI, 0.33–0.73)

MRI changes at 18 months: the median increase in lesion volume was 1% in the interferon beta-1a group compared to 16% in the placebo group

Side effects of treatment

Influenza-like syndrome: 54% of interferon beta-1a group vs 26% of placebo group

Depression: 20% of interferon beta-1a group vs 13% of placebo group

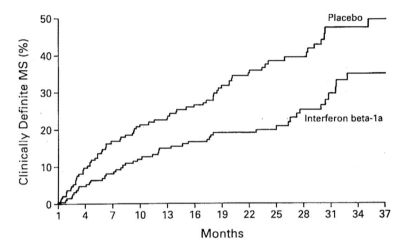

Figure 5–6. *Percentage of patients developing CDMS over 37 months was less in the treated group. (Jacobs LD et al, NEJM 343:898–904, 2000 with permission).*

TABLE 5–9. CHAMPS CONCLUSIONS

Once weekly intramuscular interferon beta-1a initiated at the time of a first clinical demyelinating event may be beneficial in patients who have MRI evidence of prior subclinical demyelination, reducing the risk of CDMS by approximately half

Interferon beta-1a is well tolerated, with no serious treatment-related adverse effects

LEBER'S STELLATE NEURORETINITIS

Leber's stellate neuroretinitis is characterized by loss of vision associated with concomitant swelling of the optic nerve and hard exudates arranged in a star configuration at the macula. Although this is primarily a retinal disorder, it is included in this section because it is frequently confused with optic neuritis.

Epidemiology and Etiology

Neuroretinitis is considered to be an infectious or immune-mediated process. Up to 50% of patients have an antecedent viral illness, usually affecting the respiratory tract, a few weeks before the onset of visual symptoms. Although neuroretinitis affects persons of all ages, it is most common in children and young adults. The vast majority of patients with neuroretinitis have no cause identified or it is associated with cat-scratch disease *(Bartonella henselae)*. Other various infections have been implicated and include: syphilis, Lyme disease, and toxoplasmosis. Some clinicians use the term neuroretinitis to refer to hypertensive retinopathy, which has both optic disc swelling and a macular star.

Clinical Characteristics

Symptoms   Painless loss of vision.

Signs

1. Visual acuity: ranges from 20/20 to light perception.
2. RAPD if unilateral or asymmetric.
3. Decreased color vision.
4. Typical fundus picture: (Figure 5–7).
   • Optic disc swelling: mild to severe.
   • Macular star and exudates deposited within Henle's layer, giving a typical star or hemistar appearance to the macula.
5. Fluorescein angiography shows leakage of dye from vessels on the disc; whereas macular vasculature is usually entirely normal.

This investigation is not necessary for the diagnosis.

Natural History

Neuroretinitis is usually a self-limiting condition, with the optic disc swelling resolving in 6 to 8 weeks. The macular star can take several months to resolve. The majority of patients regain good vision. If visual symptoms persist, the patient usually complains of metamorphopsia or blurred central vision.

Investigations

1. History of being scratched by a kitten, which maximally exposes the patient to cat scratch fever. In this circumstance, titers for *Bartonella henselae* should be drawn.
2. A swollen optic nerve and exudates, and a star figure in the macula may be seen in other conditions, for example, hypertensive optic neuropathy (see p. 62, Figure 5–20). Therefore, the patient's blood pressure should be obtained.
3. It should be noted that this fundus picture is not recognized as the equivalent of optic neuritis. It does not increase the risk of developing MS.

Treatment

Treatment depends on etiology. Antibiotic therapy is indicated for cat scratch fever. Lowering of the blood pressure is indicated for hypertensive optic neuropathy.

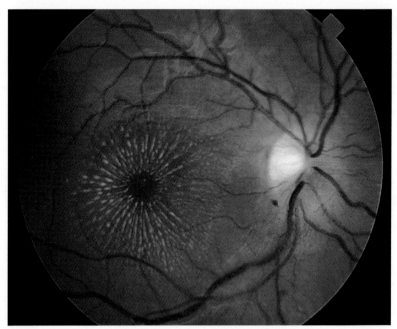

Figure 5–7. *The optic disc is swollen with nerve fiber layer edema and a hemorrhage at the 7 o'clock position off the disc. The exudates in the macula form of a star.*

SARCOID OPTIC NEUROPATHY

Sarcoidosis is a multisystem granulomatous inflammation with ocular, neurologic, and neurooph-thalmic manifestations. An optic neuropathy may develop at any time during the course of systemic sarcoidosis or it can be the initial manifestation of the disease.

Etiology

Sarcoidosis is a granulomatous inflammatory process that is identified pathologically by a noncaseating granuloma. Epithelioid and giant cells are characteristic findings on histopathologic studies.

Mechanism of Optic Nerve Involvement
The optic neuropathy of sarcoidosis is produced by one of three possible mechanisms.

1. *Compression* produced by a granuloma or by pachymeningitis (Figure 5–8).
2. *Infiltration* by inflammatory cells. Sarcoid granulomas may be seen in the optic disc (Figure 5–9).
3. *Ischemia* due to an obliterative arteritis.

Depending on the site of optic nerve involvement the neuropathy may be:

1. Unilateral or bilateral.
2. Anterior (with optic disc edema) or retro-

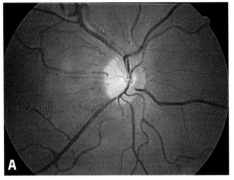
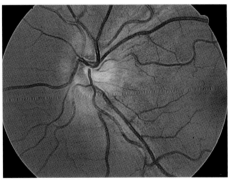
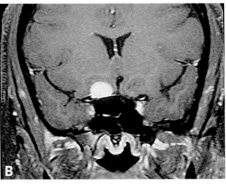

Figure 5–8. *A. Right optic nerve is pale with marked loss of the retinal nerve fiber layer. The left optic disc is congenitally anomalous but normal.* ***B.*** *MRI shows enhancing mass in the area of the planum sphenoidale compressing the right optic nerve.*

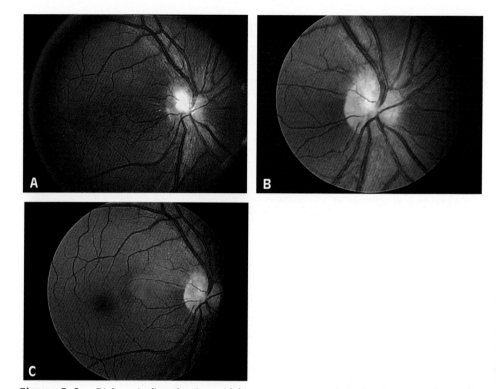

Figure 5–9. *Right optic disc of patient with biopsy proven sarcoidosis showing a granuloma of the optic disc (**A**) that disappeared after 2 years of treatment with systemic corticosteroids (**B** and **C**).*

bulbar with the optic disc appearing normal initially.

3. Optic atrophy may be the end result of any optic neuropathy.

Clinical Characteristics

Symptoms

1. Unilateral or bilateral decreased vision that is usually slowly progressive but may progress rapidly.
2. Decreased color perception.

Signs Other ocular signs of sarcoidosis are listed in Table 5–10.

1. Decreased visual acuity.
2. A RAPD if unilateral or asymmetric.

3. Acquired dyschromatopsia.
4. Central scotoma or other variations of nerve fiber bundle defects are plotted on perimetric evaluation.
5. Signs of anterior granulomatous uveitis with flare, cells, or mutton fat KP, present.
6. Optic disc may be normal, pale, swollen and hyperemic, or show the presence of a sarcoid granuloma.
7. A vitreous inflammatory reaction can be seen at times. Lesions at the level of the retinal pigment epithelium produce white areas in the fundus (Figure 5–10). The retinal changes described in the past as venous sheathing (candle wax drippings) are actually retinal or choroidal lesions that at times coalesce (Figure 5–11).
8. Non-optic nerve manifestations of sarcoidosis are listed in Table 5–11.

TABLE 5–10. OTHER OCULAR FEATURES OF SARCOIDOSIS

Lids and anterior segment
  Lupus pernio: eyelids involved with purple sarcoid indurating rash
  Lacrimal gland infiltration and enlargement
  Band keratopathy
  Conjunctival follicles
  Episcleritis and scleritis with nodules
Uvea
  Anterior uveitis: usually granulomatous with mutton fat keratic precipitates (a frequent finding)
  Pars planitis
  Vitritis
Posterior segment
  Choroiditis with yellow or white nodules
  Retinal neovascularization
  Choroidal granulomas

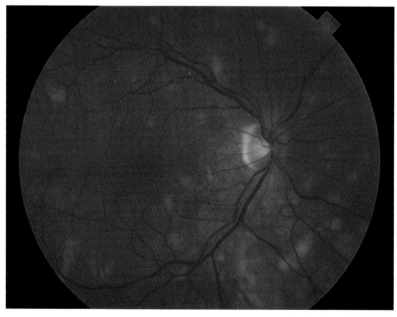

Figure 5–10. *White lesions in the posterior pole at the level of the retinal pigment epithelium.* (Courtesy of Tamara Vrabek, MD.)

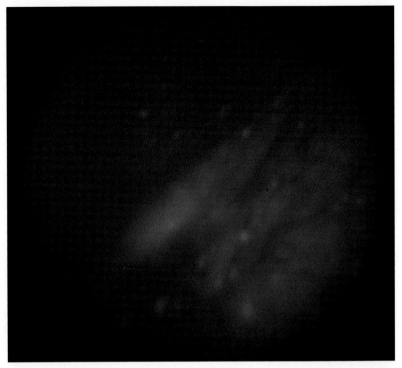

Figure 5–11. *Retinal pigment epithelium atrophy that may coalesce to form "candle wax spots" in the fundus of patients with sarcoidosis.* (Courtesy of Tamara Vrabek, MD.)

TABLE 5–11. OTHER NEUROOPHTHALMIC MANIFESTATIONS OF SARCOIDOSIS

Afferent visual pathway
  Chiasmal involvement:
    Visual field defects: bitemporal hemianopia, junctional scotoma, and bilateral optic nerve involvement
    Postchiasmal visual pathway: the pattern of the visual field defects depends on the area of the visual pathway that is involved; mechanism of damage can include compression, infiltration, or vascular occlusion related to angiitis
Efferent visual pathway
  Abducens nerve palsy most common; may be unilateral or bilateral
  Supranuclear gaze palsy and ocular flutter have been described
Pupils (uncommon)
  Tonic pupil
Orbital involvement
  Orbital mass (granuloma)
  Infiltration of extraocular muscles
  Diffuse infiltration of orbit

Investigation

1. MRI will show enhancement of the optic nerve or the portion of the anterior visual pathway that is involved (Figure 5–12). The meninges may be thickened and show abnormal enhancement.
2. Serum ACE levels may be abnormally high.
3. Chest x-ray or imaging will often show hilar adenopathy or pulmonary nodules or infiltrates.
4. Pulmonary function studies often reveal restrictive pulmonary disease.
5. Gallium scan documents involvement of the lung and lacrimal glands in many patients.
6. Definitive diagnosis is established by biopsy. Tissue is usually obtained from the enlarged hilar lymph nodes via bronchoscopy or from the lacrimal glands if they appear involved by the process (Figure 5–13). Blind conjunctival biopsy has a very low yield, while biopsy of a conjunctival lesion (granuloma) visible on the slit lamp examination has a much higher yield.

Treatment

1. Corticosteroids are the mainstay of treatment in this disorder. They should be given systemically for the optic neuropathy.
2. If uveitis coexists, it should be treated with a topical or periocular corticosteroid.
3. If corticosteroids fail to halt or reverse the process, agents such as methotrexate should be tried.

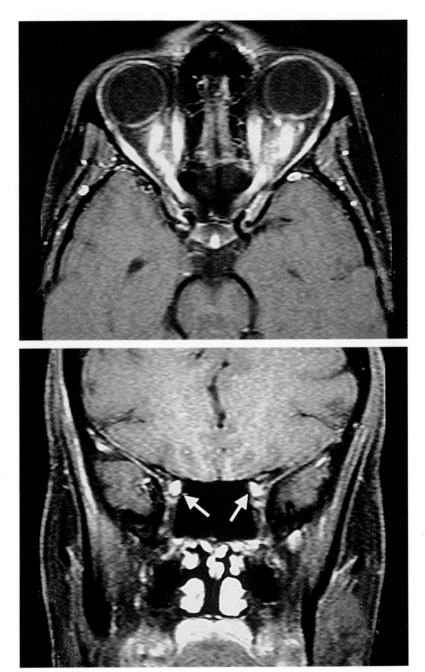

Figure 5–12. *MRI axial (top) and coronal (bottom) of patient with sarcoidosis and decreased vision bilaterally showing enhancement of both optic nerves along their entire course.*

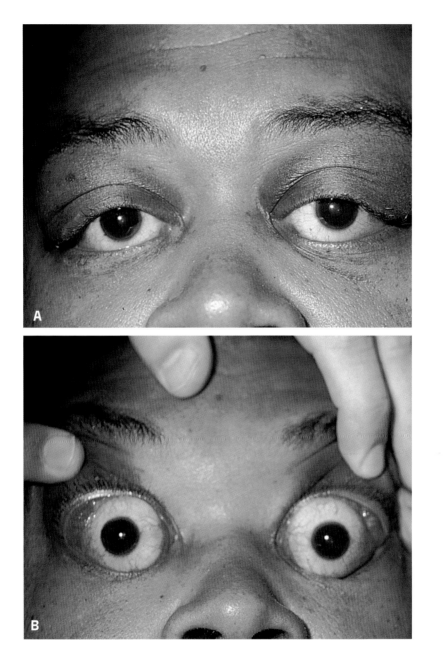

Figure 5–13. *A. Sarcoidosis producing fullness bilaterally in the area of the lacrimal glands. B. Elevation of the lids shows prolapse of the enlarged lacrimal glands.*

SYPHILITIC OPTIC NEUROPATHY

Abnormalities of the optic nerve may be encountered in both secondary and tertiary syphilis.

Etiology

Syphilis

Clinical Characteristics

The general ocular signs of syphilis are listed in Table 5–12.

Symptoms

1. Decreased vision, which may be unilateral or bilateral.
2. Decreased color perception.

**TABLE 5–12. OCULAR MANIFES-
TATIONS OF
SYPHILIS**

Primary: chancre on eyelid
Secondary
 Uveitis
  Panuveitis
  Choroiditis
  Choroidoretinitis
 Optic neuritis
 Retinitis and retinal vasculitis
 Papilledema
 Anterior segment
  Episcleritis
  Scleritis
  Dacryoadenitis
  Dacryocystitis
  Interstitial keratitis
  Iris papules and gumma
Tertiary
 Optic neuropathy
 Argyll Robertson pupil
 Interstitial keratitis
 Chronic uveitis
 Ocular motor neuropathies, especially CN III

Signs

1. Central scotomas.
2. A RAPD if unilateral or asymmetric.
3. At times, a vitreous cellular reaction can exist, especially with papillitis and in HIV-positive patients
4. Neuroretinitis can occur in patients with secondary and tertiary syphilis. In secondary syphilis, it can occur as part of syphilitic meningitis and may be either a unilateral isolated phenomenon (with or without uveitis) or bilateral.
5. Meningitis produces involvement of other cranial nerves, or signs of meningeal irritation.

The syphilitic patient, in addition, may manifest the following optic nerve abnormalities.

1. *Optic perineuritis* (perioptic neuritis): the optic disc is swollen but visual acuity is normal and there are no other clinical signs of an optic neuropathy. This is usually a manifestation of secondary syphilis.
2. *Papillitis:* this anterior optic neuritis may be indistinguishable from demyelinating optic neuritis (Figure 5–14). It usually produces rapid visual loss. It may be seen in both secondary and tertiary syphilis.
3. *Neuroretinitis:* may be accompanied by vitritis and is encountered in both secondary or tertiary syphilis.
4. *Retrobulbar optic neuritis:* appears as a typical optic neuropathy except the visual loss may be rapid and profound in secondary syphilis. In tertiary disease it is a slowly progressive phenomenon.
5. *Papilledema:* may accompany the meningitis in secondary and tertiary disease. Its appearance may be confused with optic

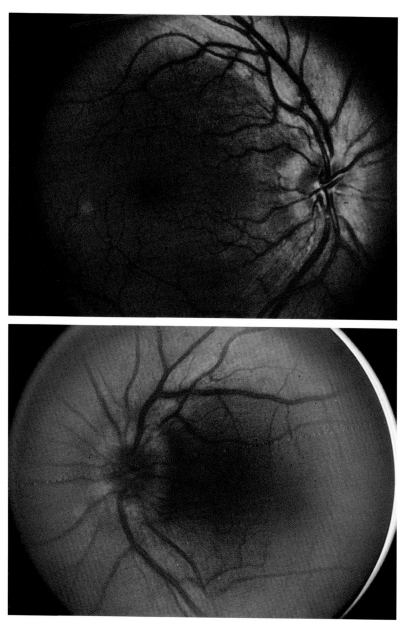

Figure 5–14. *Patient with bilateral papillitis due to syphilis. The optic disc returned to normal after completion of intravenous penicillin therapy*

perineuritis until lumbar puncture documents increased intracranial pressure.

Diagnosis

The best method to prove a syphilitic infection is to demonstrate the spirocete in a tissue biopsy or CSF. This is not usually feasible so indirect methods of testing for syphilis are routinely employed.

The serologic tests for syphilis are listed in Table 5–13. Specific testing recommendations appear in Table 5–14.

Treatment

It is strongly advised that staging and treatment of syphilis be conducted by, or in consultation with, an infectious disease specialist. However, a general overview of the indications for and the methods of treatment are as follows.

Indications for treatment:

1. FTA-ABS positive and VDRL negative
    - If appropriate past treatment cannot be documented.
    - If active syphilitic signs and abnormal CSF.
    - Concurrent HIV: these patients may have negative FTA-ABS and VDRL (diagnosis is then made on clinical grounds).
2. FTA-ABS positive and VDRL positive
    - If appropriate past treatment cannot be documented.
    - If previous VDRL titer (>1:8) did not decrease fourfold within 1 year of appropriate treatment.
    - If previous titer is not available, present titer greater than 1:4, and treatment was more than several years ago.

TABLE 5–13.   TESTS FOR SYPHILIS

Treponemal Tests
Use:
  High specificity and sensitivity in all stages of syphilis
  Once reactive, these tests do not revert to normal
  Used for confirming diagnosis of syphilis
  Used routinely for suspected late syphilis
Tests
  Immunofluorescence: FTA-ABS: fluorescent treponemal antibody
  Hemagglutination
    MHA-TP: microhemagglutination treponemal test for syphilis
    HATTS: hemagglutination treponemal test
    TPHA: widely used in Canada and Europe, but not available in the United States
Nontreponemal (Reagin) Tests
Use
  Initial screening or to quantitate the serum reagin antibody titer, but there are significant false negatives in primary, latent or late syphilis
  Reflects activity of disease: eg, a rise in titers seen between primary and secondary syphilis; persistent fall in titers following treatment provides evidence of an adequate response to therapy
Tests
  VDRL: Venereal Disease Research Laboratories test
    Advantages: standard test used for CSF; less expensive
    Disadvantage: uses heated serum; reagent must be prepared fresh daily
  RPR: Rapid plasma reagin
    Advantages: easy to perform; uses unheated serum; test of choice for rapid serologic diagnosis
    Disadvantage: more expensive than VDRL

TABLE 5–14. CSF TESTING IN SYPHILITIC OPTIC NEUROPATHY

Indications for lumbar puncture
  Seropositive patient with neurologic or neuroophthalmic signs and symptoms
  All patients with untreated syphilis of unknown duration
  HIV-positive patients who are also seropositive
Test to perform
  CSF VDRL
    Very specific if fluid not contaminated with blood
    Low sensitivity: may be nonreactive in progressive symptomatic syphilis
  CSF protein, cell count

Regimen of treatment:

Neurosyphilis may be diagnosed in the presence of a positive serum FTA-ABS and either:

1. CSF-VDRL positive
2. Greater than 5 WBC/mm^3 in CSF
3. CSF protein > 45 mg/dL

Treatment consists of:

1. Intravenous aqueous crystalline penicillin G 2 to 4 million U, q4hr, for 10 to 14 days, followed by intramuscular benzathine PCN, 2.4 million U weekly for 3 weeks.

2. If the CSF is normal, only the IM benzathine PCN, 2.4 million U weekly for 3 weeks is required.
3. There is an indication that the dosage of penicillin should be higher in HIV-positive patients.

Follow-up:

Patients with neurosyphilis need repeated lumbar punctures every 6 months until the white cell count returns to normal. If it does not decrease, retreatment may be indicated.

NONARTERITIC ANTERIOR ISCHEMIC OPTIC NEUROPATHY

Nonarteritic anterior ischemic optic neuropathy (NAION) is a common disorder characterized by painless loss of vision associated with optic disc swelling. Its name indicates that it is not caused by GCA.

Pathogenesis and Etiology

NAION is thought to be the result of vascular insufficiency in the posterior ciliary circulation affecting the distal optic nerve. The incidence of NAION is between 2 to 10 per 100,000 persons over the age of 50 years. The average age of onset is between 55 to 65 (range 40 to 70) years, although it is becoming more frequently diagnosed in younger patients with known risk factors. Risk factors that are thought to be important include:

1. Small cup-to-disc ratio and small optic discs (also referred to as congenitally anomalous discs or "discs at risk") (Figure 5–15). This is probably the most important risk factor associated with NAION.
2. Hypertension.
3. Diabetes mellitus.
4. Hypercholesterolemia.
5. Other vascular risk factors: conditions associated with small vessel disease and coagulopathies may be important, although the evidence is not conclusive.
6. Following profound blood loss that may be spontaneous or as a result of surgery, or severe hypotension.
7. Post-cataract surgery.
9. Optic disc drusen appear to predispose to NAION.

Clinical Characteristics

Symptoms Patients present with painless loss of vision, although some may be asymptomatic. The level of visual loss can vary from 20/20 with a visual field defect to light perception. It would be very unusual for NAION to result in no light perception vision.

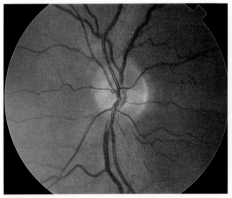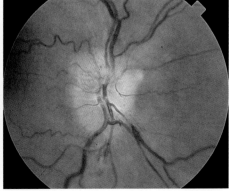

Figure 5–15. *Right eye (left) has a "disc at risk." The left disc (right) is elevated with retinal nerve fiber layer edema especially on its superior portion.*

Signs

1. Decreased visual acuity. In the Ischemic Optic Neuropathy Decompression Trial (IONDT), approximately one-half of the patients had initial visual acuity better than 20/64 and one-third had worse than 20/200.
2. Relative afferent papillary defect. An RAPD will be present unless there is optic nerve or significant retinal pathology in the contralateral eye.
3. Dyschromatopsia. The degree of decreased color vision is usually proportional to the level of visual acuity loss, unlike optic neuritis in which the color vision is usually disproportionately affected.
4. Anterior visual pathway field defect. The most common visual field defect is altitudinal in character, although any optic nerve defect may be seen.
5. Disc edema. (Figure see 5–15) The swelling of the optic disc is either diffuse or sectoral. The swelling is usually hyperemic more than pale, with flame-shaped hemorrhages occurring commonly. The optic disc edema occurs before or concurrent with visual loss. The diagnosis of AION may not be made in the presence of a normal optic disc.
6. Disc at risk in the contralateral eye.

Diagnosis and Investigations

The diagnosis is a clinical one and may be made when patients have a swollen, hyperemic optic nerve, usually with peripapillary hemorrhages and signs of an optic neuropathy. Clinical features suggesting other causes of an anterior optic neuropathy (GCA, inflammatory optic neuropathies) should be excluded.

Giant cell arteritis needs to be excluded as the cause of AION in all patients over the age of 55 years. This involves a thorough history and examination to identify other symptoms and signs of GCA (see Chapter 5) and performing an ESR and/or a C reactive problem (CRP).

Other investigations that could be considered useful are aimed at identifying underlying vascular risk factors (blood pressure, fasting glucose, cardiology assessment), although there is no evidence that controlling these risk factors prevents another episode from developing.

The edema of NAION resolves within 6 to 8 weeks. If the disc edema is present for greater than 2 months, further investigations to identify another cause for the optic neuropathy should be undertaken.

Course

The visual dysfunction may be maximal at onset or it may worsen over days or even weeks in up to 35% of patients. The IONDT investigators claim that approximately 40% of patients will recover three or more lines of vision. The disc edema resolves over several weeks, with optic atrophy associated with attenuation of the arterioles at the disc margin replacing the edema. The estimated risk of developing NAION in the contralateral eye ranges from 12% up to 40%. There is less than a 5% risk of having a second event in the same eye.

Treatment

No therapy has been proven to be effective in NAION.

GIANT CELL ARTERITIS

Giant cell (temporal, cranial) arteritis is a frequently encountered systemic necrotizing vasculitis of medium and large arteries that has several of the most important neuroophthalmologic manifestations encountered. However, it still presents a challenge as to its cause and the optimum treatment.

Incidence

The incidence of GCA in the United States is stated to be 17.8/100,000 in men and 24.2/100,000 in woman over 50 years of age on the basis of a study performed in Olmsted County, Minnesota. However, because the incidence of GCA in non-Caucasians, including the Hispanic, African American, and Asian populations is much less, its true national incidence may be less. Some reports also describe a seasonal variation in the occurrence of GCA, while other investigators have found no such fluctuation.

Age is an all-important factor. All the incidence statistics are calculated for patients over age 50 years. It is extraordinarily rare for GCA to occur in patients younger than 50 years of age, and most patients afflicted with this disorder actually are in their sixties or older.

Pathogenesis and Etiology

The exact cause of GCA is not known. It is apparent that GCA is a genetic disorder, as evidenced by its increased incidence in Northern Europeans and their descendents in this country, as well as the high association of HLA-DRB1.

Although the initial trigger of this immunologic disorder is unknown, it produces an influx of CD4-type T cells via the vaso vasorum into the tunica adventitia. These T cells produce IFN-γ, which causes obliteration of the vessel lumen. Macrophages also enter via the vaso vasorum and they secrete interleukin-6 (IL-6) and IL-1β. These macrophages in the media of the arterial wall secrete metalloproteinases, which are enzymes that can digest arterial wall components. This causes a liberation of smooth muscle cells, which migrate toward the lumen causing intimal hyperplasia. Thus, the major process that produces ischemia in GCA is not destruction of the arterial wall, but luminal obstruction caused by a hyperplastic reaction of the intima. This hyperplasia of the intima in response to an antigen-driven immune response requires new capillary formation in all three layers (media, adventitia, interna) to support this new tissue. These inflamed arteries produce platelet-derived growth factors (PDGF A and B), whose expression correlates with luminal obstruction. These factors are produced by macrophages and giant cells found at the media–intima border. Stenotic lesions also have a higher concentration of vascular endothelial growth factor (VEGF).

Clinical Characteristics

Giant cell arteritis is a disorder that is closely related to the systemic disorder polymyalgia rheumatica (PMR). About 50% of the people who have biopsy-proven GCA will have PMR. A form of GCA termed *occult* presents with sudden visual loss without the patient having any of the systemic signs or symptoms that are normally associated with GCA and PMR. It is estimated that approximately 20% of patients with biopsy-proven GCA may have the occult form.

Symptoms

1. Visual loss. It is sudden and usually profound.

2. Diplopia. This is estimated to be the presenting symptom of GCA in approximately 15% of patients.
3. Transient visual loss. This may be in one or both eyes and can last from minutes to hours.
4. Headache. Usually the headache is of new onset.
5. Scalp tenderness. Patients may localize this to the area over the superficial temporal artery or it may be more generalized. They will frequently complain of difficulty combing their hair, wearing their glasses, or even resting the side of their head on a pillow.
6. Jaw claudication. Chewing produces pain in the masseter muscle due to ischemia. This symptom is highly suggestive of GCA.
7. Constitutional symptoms. Patients have loss of appetite, weight loss, and asthenia.
8. Polymyalgia rheumatica:This is characterized by pain and stiffness in the proximal muscle groups that is worse in the morning and after activity.

Signs A variety of ocular problems may occur with GCA, but the most distressing is visual loss, which is estimated to occur in approximately 50% of GCA patients. The causes of visual loss in GCA are:

1. Arteritic anterior ischemic optic neuropathy (A-AION): A-AION is an infarction within the prelaminar and laminar portion of the optic nerve due to vasoobliterative occlusion of the short posterior ciliary arteries. It is estimated that A-AION is the cause of visual loss in approximately 50% of GCA patients. The A-AION of GCA has a characteristic appearance. The optic disc is infarcted and has a chalk white color, which is usually total instead of segmental. Often, areas of ischemia, such as retinal whitening continuous with the optic disc or cotton wool infarcts in the retina, will accompany AION (Figure 5–16) Retinal ischemia in the presence of AION is overwhelming circumstantial evidence that the cause of the AION is GCA. The visual loss in A-AION usually is much more profound than in NAION. Vision can be severely affected to hand motion and no light perception, levels of visual dysfunction that are infrequently encountered with NAION. Arteritic AION also tends to be

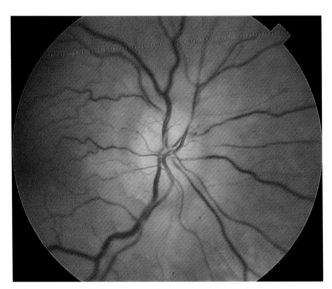

Figure 5–16. *The optic disc is infarcted. It has a chalk-like color. There are some nerve fiber layer hemorrhages. Inferiorly, there is some extension of the infarction into the retina characteristic of giant cell arteritis.*

bilateral. It can affect the contralateral eye, usually within days or weeks, even if treatment is administered. Thus, the diagnosis of GCA and the institution of the appropriate treatment become critical before the second eye is involved. Following resolution of the optic disc edema, the optic disc appearance is different in A-AION than in NAION. While the latter presents with sectoral or total pallor, the A-AION disc typically shows cupping.

2. Retinal artery occlusion: central retinal artery occlusion (CRAO) (more rarely, branch retinal artery occlusion) is a less frequent cause of visual loss in GCA. Clinically, it presents in a manner similar to other retinal artery occlusions with sudden visual loss and the appearance of retinal whitening. The appearance of CRAO in an elderly patient who does not have visible embolic material in the retinal arterioles must raise the suspicion of GCA.

3. Posterior ischemic optic neuropathy (PION): infarction of the optic disc posterior to the laminar cribrosa may occur in GCA. This will result in sudden visual loss, which may be unilateral or bilateral, and initially the optic disc will appear normal. Subsequently, the disc will become pale. This is an unusual manifestation of GCA, but overall GCA is one of the more frequent causes of PION

4. Choroidal ischemia: at times, the fundus appears normal or minimally involved for the profound degree of visual loss. Fluorescein angiography may reveal marked deficiency of blood flowing to the choroid (Figure 5–17).

5. Ocular ischemic syndrome: this is an unusual presentation for GCA, but the diagnosis must be kept in mind in patients who present with decreased vision, ocular hypotony, and anterior segment inflammation. This syndrome is due to involvement of the ophthalmic artery by the arteritic process.

6. Ocular misalignment: double vision may be caused by infarction of the extraocular muscles, CN III, IV, or VI, or by infarction in the brain stem, causing ocular misalignment as part of the overall stroke syndrome.

7. Abnormal superficial temporal arteries: they may be indurated, prominent, without a pulse and painful (Figure 5–18).

Other systemic problems secondary to arteritis that may be associated with GCA include:

1. Brain stem strokes

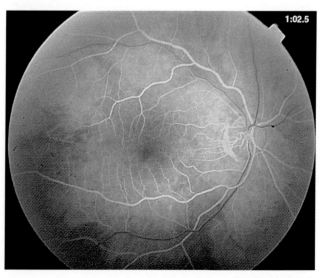

Figure 5–17. *Fluorescein angiogram showing delayed choroidal filling after 1 minute.*

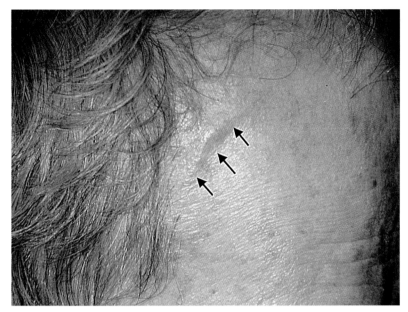

Figure 5–18. *Patient with giant cell arteritis showing indurated nonpulsatile tender superficial temporal artery* (arrows).

2. Dissecting aneurysm
3. Aortic incompetence
4. Myocardial infarction
6. Infarction of other organs: bowel, kidney

Diagnosis

Laboratory tests are used to assist in the diagnosis GCA.

1. The ESR is the time-honored test for GCA and is usually elevated. It is, however, not specific and may be elevated when GCA is not present and be normal when it is. We prefer the Westergren method because it is more accurate at higher levels. We use the formula of age/2 in men and age + 10/2 in women as the normal values for the WESR.

2. The CRP is said to be a more sensitive indicator for the presence of GCA than is the ESR. It is estimated that fewer than 2 % of patients will have a temporal artery biopsy positive for GCA and have a normal CRP.

3. *Thrombocytosis*: patients with GCA will often have platelet counts greater than 400 $\times$ 10 ^{3}/uL.

4. *Intravenous fluorescein angiography* (IVFA) will often show delayed choroidal filling in patients with GCA.

5. *Ultrasonic imaging* of the superficial temporal artery using color Doppler technology has shown a characteristic dark halo, which was interpreted as being due to edema in the arteriole wall. Color Doppler will also show decreased blood flow velocity in the involved superficial temporal artery.

6. *Temporal artery biopsy* is the gold standard of the diagnosis of GCA. A positive biopsy consists of finding inflammatory mononuclear cells with destruction of the internal elastic lamina. There may be necrosis of the media and multinucleated giant cells may be present, but the diagnosis may be made in their absence (Figure 5–19). Statistics show that a unilateral negative temporal artery biopsy is excellent evidence that the patient does not have GCA. However, if the

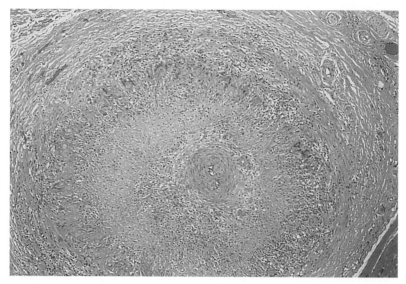

Figure 5–19. *Temporal artery biopsy specimen shows inflammation with occlusion of the arterial lumen. Multinucleated giant cells also are evident.*

clinical suspicion is high, the consequences of missing the diagnosis, even though this is statistically unlikely, are so important that the second, contralateral artery should be biopsied. It matters little whether biopsies are done simultaneously, sequentially or under frozen-section guidance. All patients suspected of having GCA should undergo temporal artery biopsy even if the clinical picture is compelling. This prevents the premature interruption of treatment when complications of steroid therapy occur. It also avoids the difficult task of trying to diagnose GCA by finding evidence of so-called "healed GCA" on temporal artery biopsy months after treatment has begun.

Treatment

There is only one treatment for GCA and that is systemic corticosteroids. The exact dosage of corticosteroids required to prevent visual loss and the duration of the treatment regimen are unknown. The primary goal of treatment in a patient who has GCA is to prevent visual loss in either eye if the diagnosis is made before visual loss occurs, or in the fellow eye if the diagnosis is established after unilateral visual loss. The second goal of therapy, that is, reversal of visual loss, is more controversial. There are no prospective randomized studies that have investigated the efficacy of different corticosteroid treatment regimens in reversing visual loss.

We recommend that patients who have suffered a fixed visual deficit be admitted and treated with 250 mg of intravenous methylprednisolone q6hr. During the 3 days of hospitalization and treatment, temporal artery biopsy should be performed, and if it is positive, the patient is discharged on oral prednisone that averages 1 mg/kg/day. Patients who do not have visual loss may be treated as an outpatient with oral prednisone pending results of temporal artery biopsy. *All patients suspected of having GCA should be treated with corticosteroids while diagnostic information, including the results of the temporal artery biopsy, is being collected.*

HYPERTENSIVE OPTIC NEUROPATHY

Hypertensive optic neuropathy is characterized by bilateral optic disc swelling in hypertensive patients.

Epidemiology and Etiology

Hypertension is usually significant, with diastolic pressures over 100 mm Hg.

Clinical Characteristics

Symptoms Decreased vision is the only symptom. The disc edema may be noted on routine eye or medical evaluation.

Signs

1. Decreased acuity may be on the basis of optic nerve or retinal involvement.
2. Constricted visual fields.
3. A RAPD if asymmetric.
4. Swollen optic discs (Figure 5–20).
5. Fundus changes characteristic of systemic hypertension with arteriolar narrowing, A-V crossing changes, retinal exudates, or retinal/choroidal infarcts.

Management and Therapy

Lowering of blood pressure. It is important not to lower the blood pressure too rapidly to avoid infarction of the optic nerves.

Differential Diagnosis

1. Papilledema
2. Ischemic optic neuropathy
3. Uremic papillopathy

Special Comments

Hypertensive optic neuropathy is thought to be a form of ischemic optic neuropathy. However, there are instances in which hypertensive optic neuropathy is due to increased intracranial pressure. When this is the cause of the optic disc swelling, patients usually have symptoms of diffuse encephalopathy.

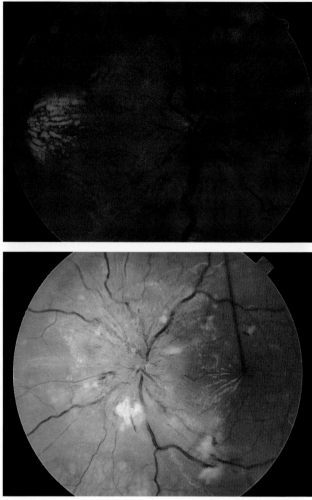

Figure 5–20. *Bilateral swollen optic discs with retinal infarcts and exudates in the form of a hemimacular star figure. The patient's blood pressure was 210/130 mm Hg.*

DIABETIC PAPILLOPATHY

Diabetic papillopathy is unilateral or bilateral optic disc swelling that occurs in patients with diabetes mellitus. It is thought to be an atypical form of NAION.

Epidemiology and Etiology

Diabetic papillopathy was initially described in type 1 diabetes mellitus, but occurs in both type 1 and type 2 diabetes mellitus. The cause of the disc swelling is not known.

Clinical Characteristics

Symptoms   Visual loss is usually present and is the only symptom.

Signs

1. Optic disc swelling, which may be unilateral or bilateral. More peripapillary hemorrhages are present than in NAION (Figure 5–21).
2. A RAPD if visual loss is asymmetric or unilateral.
3. Visual field defects including central scotomas, arcuate visual field defect.
4. Diabetic retinopathy is usually present, although rarely it may be absent.
5. Macular edema is frequently present.

Clinical Course

The clinical course of diabetic papillopathy is usually benign, with many patients experiencing complete recovery of vision. The disc edema may take months to disappear.

Treatment

None is required other than control of the diabetic state.

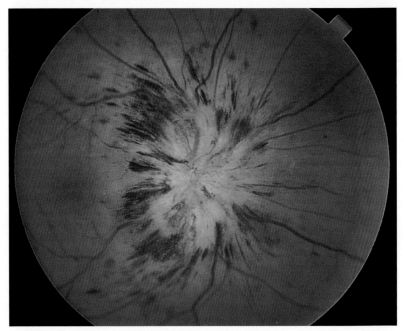

Figure 5–21. *Optic disc is elevated with numerous peripapillary hemorrhages. Diabetic retinopathy and macular edema are also present.*

RADIATION OPTIC NEUROPATHY

A unilateral or bilateral optic neuropathy may develop following radiation therapy.

Epidemiology and Etiology

This optic neuropathy usually occurs in patients with intracranial, skull-base, or paranasal sinus tumors who have undergone radiation therapy where the optic nerves are included in the radiation field. A dose above 6000 cGy with daily fractions of about 200 cGy is necessary to produce radiation induced optic neuropathy. It is also known to occur following radiation for thyroid orbitopathy in patients with pre-existing diabetes mellitus. It should be remembered that lower doses of radiation might produce radiation optic neuropathy if given at the same time as chemotherapy, which seems to potentiate the effect of the radiation on the optic nerve.

The exact mechanism is not known but is presumed to be radiation-induced damage to the vascular endothelial cells that subsequently results in vascular occlusion and necrosis. It usually presents as a retrobulbar optic neuropathy, although rarely, it may present as an anterior optic neuropathy with a swollen optic nerve.

Clinical Characteristics

Symptoms Visual loss occurs acutely and progresses until most or all vision is lost in one or both eyes. Visual loss usually occurs an average of 18 months following the radiation therapy, but may occur within the first year, and has been reported to occur after 20 years.

Signs

1. Decreased visual acuity.
2. Visual field defects of optic nerve or chiasmal origin.
3. Initially, the optic discs appear normal, but subsequently become pale.

Diagnosis

The diagnosis is established clinically in a patient who has received the appropriate amount of radiation and in whom other causes of visual loss have been excluded. The differential diagnosis includes recurrence of the initial tumor, secondary empty sella syndrome with optic nerve and chiasmal prolapse, radiation-induced parasellar tumor, and arachnoiditis.

CT scans are normal and there is no enhancement with contrast. However, T1-weighted gadolinium-enhanced MRI will show marked enhancement of the optic nerves, optic chiasm, and possibly the optic tracts (see Figure 6–11, p. 129). The enhancement resolves when the visual function stabilizes. Unenhanced T1- and T2-weighted image will show no abnormality.

Treatment

This is a vascular necrosis that causes visual loss. Various treatments have been championed, including high-dose corticosteroids, alone or combined with hyperbaric oxygen treatment. Their effectiveness is somewhat doubtful.

Radiation necrosis of the brain appears to respond to anticoagulation therapy. There are no studies, however, to indicate that this treatment is effective in radiation-induced optic neuropathy. However, it should be tried since the ultimate outcome is usually blindness.

Prognosis

Almost half of all patients will have a final visual outcome of no light perception despite various treatment attempts. Those who maintain some vision will have VA worse than 20/200.

AMIODARONE OPTIC NEUROPATHY

Amiodarone optic neuropathy has been attributed to the systemic administration of the cardiac antiarrhythmic drug amiodarone.

Epidemiology and Etiology

Amiodarone-associated optic neuropathy is thought to occur in approximately 1 to 2% of patients taking the drug. The exact cause of the optic neuropathy is not known. Lipid inclusions characteristic of amiodarone have been found in one optic nerve studied histopathologically. This supports the concept that amiodarone can affect the optic nerve.

Clinical Characteristics

Symptoms Decreased vision is insidious in onset and is slowly progressive as long as the drug is taken. Some patients may have no visual complaints.

Signs

1. Optic disc swelling is bilateral (Figure 5–22). Cases of unilateral involvement have been reported but these may be instances of NAION in patients who happen to be taking amiodarone.
2. Decreased visual acuity which is usually not worse than 20/200.
3. Visual field deficits of the optic nerve variety.
4. A RAPD if visual deficits are asymmetric.
5. Acquired dyschromatopsia.
6. Vortex keratopathy: whorl-like opacities in the corneal endothelium that do not produce decreased vision but are present in patients taking amiodarone.

Differential Diagnosis

1. *Papilledema:* because of the bilateral disc elevation. However, the loss of vision in the absence of chronic disc changes eliminates papilledema as a possible diagnosis.
2. *Ischemic optic neuropathy* is the entity most often confused with amiodarone optic neuropathy. A comparison of their differentiating characteristics is seen in Table 5–15.

Investigations

No investigations prove the existence of amiodarone-induced optic neuropathy. The presence of optic disc edema in a patient taking amiodarone is grounds to suspect this diagnosis.

Treatment

In any patient with suspected amiodarone-induced optic neuropathy, the drug should be discontinued if another form of treatment for the cardiac disorder is available. No other treatment to reverse the optic neuropathy exists.

We recommend that the prescribing physician discontinue the amiodarone if this is medically feasible. The patient is reexamined within 6 to 8 weeks. If the disc edema is still evident, the diagnosis of amiodarone-induced optic neuropathy is made.

Clinical Course

After discontinuing the medication, the optic disc edema slowly resolves and in approximately one-third of patients, visual function re-

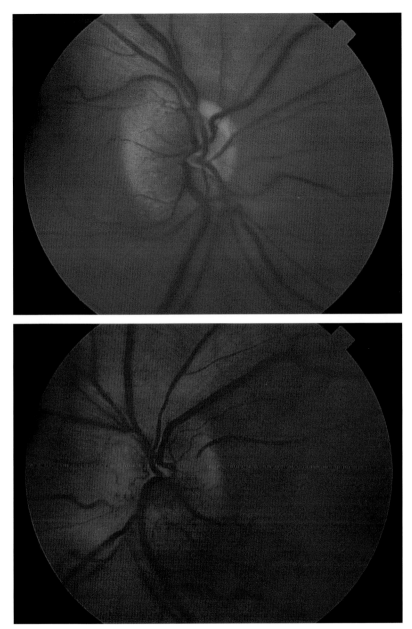

Figure 5–22. *Bilateral optic disc edema with decreased vision and visual field loss in a patient taking amiodarone. The disc edema subsided with return of visual function 4 months after the medication was discontinued.*

TABLE 5–15. AMIODARONE-INDUCED OPTIC NEUROPATHY VS NAION

	Amiodarone	NAION
Onset of symptoms	Insidious	Acute
Laterality	Bilateral, simultaneous	Unilateral, if bilateral, usually sequential
Resolution of edema	Months	6–8 weeks

covers as the optic disc edema subsides. Vision usually stabilizes in the other patients.

Special Features

There is controversy as to whether amiodarone-induced optic neuropathy exists as a diagnosis *sui generis,* or whether these patients actually have NAION and happen to be taking amiodarone. It is difficult at times to make a distinction between the two entities. We believe the major differentiating factor that distinguishes between the two is the time to resolution of the optic disc swelling. The disc edema of NAION will resolve within 6 to 8 weeks, whereas the edema of amiodarone-induced optic neuropathy will take many more weeks to months to resolve.

NUTRITIONAL DEFICIENCY AND TOXIC OPTIC NEUROPATHIES

NUTRITIONAL OPTIC NEUROPATHY

In the past, nutritional optic neuropathy was referred to as tobacco alcohol amblyopia because it was believed that the combined toxic effect of those two agents produced this optic neuropathy. It is now accepted that this is a nutritional optic neuropathy.

Etiology and Epidemiology

1. A specific nutritional deficit has not been identified.
2. These patients ordinarily do smoke and drink to excess and do have a very poor diet, usually lacking in fresh vegetables.
3. There is a suspicion that the cyanide contained in tobacco may contribute to the production of this optic neuropathy in smokers.

Clinical Presentation

The hallmark of the optic neuropathy due to either nutritional deficiencies or toxic exposure is bilateral, simultaneous, painless visual loss.

Symptoms

1. Progressive loss of vision
   • Bilateral: although may be somewhat asymmetric, particularly in the early stages.
   • Rate of decline: may be quite rapid.
   • Extent of visual loss: variable, but central acuity is usually better than count fingers.
2. Acquired dyschromatopsia: usually present early and may be the initial symptom.

Signs

1. Bilateral central or centrocecal scotomas, usually with intact peripheral visual fields,

are the hallmark of toxic optic neuropathies.
2. Pupillary reaction usually is sluggish.
3. Absence of a RAPD: because of the bilateral and symmetric involvement of the optic nerves.
4. Optic atrophy, involving mostly the papillomacular area of the disc, appears later in the disease course (Figure 5–23). Initially, the optic disc may be normal or hyperemic.

Diagnosis

1. Detailed history: with particular attention to dietary intake, smoking habits, alcohol consumption, and other medical conditions of relevance. Other disorders that may produce bilateral visual loss are listed in Table 5–16.
2. Physical examination seeking other signs of nutritional deficiencies.
3. Neuroimaging: MRI with intravenous injection of gadolinium DTPA is usually prudent to exclude an underlying compressive lesion of both optic nerves or the optic chiasm.
4. Special investigations
   • Vitamin B$_{12}$ level: to exclude pernicious anemia.
   • Red blood cell folate level may be performed but may be normal.

Treatment

1. Discontinue alcohol consumption and use of tobacco.
2. Improve dietary intake, specifically with green and yellow vegetables.
3. Prescribe thiamine 100 mg po bid and folate 1.0 mg po daily.
4. Vitamin B$_{12}$ injections are recommended by some. The hydroxycobalamine form should be administered.

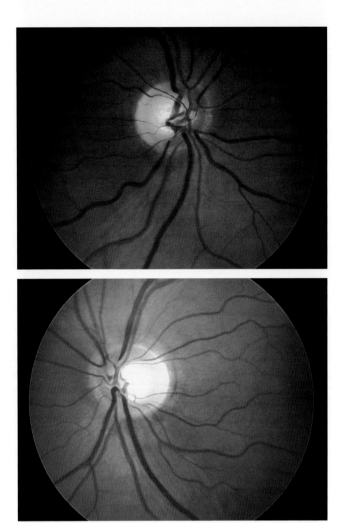

Figure 5–23. *Bilateral temporal optic disc pallor with decreased vision and central scotomas in a patient with presumed nutritional deficiency optic neuropathy.*

The goal of treatment is usually to prevent further visual loss. Most patients present when their optic discs are atrophic and they have well-established visual loss. If patients are diagnosed and treated early, when the optic discs are normal or even hyperemic, there is a possibility of return of some visual function.

TABLE 5–16. DIFFERENTIAL DIAGNOSIS OF BILATERAL VISUAL LOSS

Macular disease
Compressive or infiltrative lesions of the optic nerve or chiasm
Dominant optic atrophy
Leber's optic neuropathy
Conversion disorder or malingering.

SPECIFIC DEFICIENCY OPTIC NEUROPATHIES

Vitamin B12 Deficiency

Cause

1. Pernicious anemia: is the most common cause.
   - Autoimmune disorder most commonly seen in middle aged and elderly Caucasians.
   - Vitamin B_{12} is poorly absorbed from the ileum because the parietal cells of the gastric mucosa do not produce intrinsic factor.
   - Megaloblastic anemia.
   - Neurologic symptoms: subacute combined degeneration.
2. Poor diet: usually in strict vegans.
3. Other causes of impaired absorption:
   - gastrointestinal surgery,
   - intestinal disease,
   - diphyllobothriasis, and
   - intestinal tapeworms.

Treatment

Intramuscular injections of hydroxycobalamin (not cyanocobalamin).

Thiamine Deficiency

The evidence that thiamine deficiency can produce an optic neuropathy is inconclusive, al-though patients who have nutritional optic neuropathy may also be thiamine deficient. It is still recommended that patients with nutritional optic neuropathy be screened for thiamine and folic acid deficiency and treated.

Toxic Optic Neuropathies

For a detailed list, see Tables 5–17 and 5–18.

Methanol

Clinical Presentation

The patient usually has accidentally ingested methanol because it was mistaken for or substituted for ethyl alcohol.

Clinical Characteristics

Symptoms

1. Nausea and vomiting: occur early after ingestion.
2. Respiratory distress, abdominal discomfort, and headache: after 18 to 48 hours. The patient also may have confusion, generalized weakness, and drowsiness.
3. Metabolic acidosis.
4. Visual loss is acute and severe most commonly, but visual acuity may be reduced to any level. Central or centrocecal scotomas are characteristic if some vision is preserved.

TABLE 5–17.   TOXIC OPTIC NEUROPATHIES

Agent	Usage	Systemic Association	Optic Neuropathy	Other neuro-ophthalmic Findings
Ethylene glycol	Automobile antifreeze	Nausea, vomiting, abdominal pain, coma	Mild to profound visual loss.	Nystagmus, ophthalmoplegia
Halogenated hydroxyquinolones	Amebacidal drugs	Abdominal discomfort, parasthesias, dysethesias	Dyschromatopsia early finding	Subacute myelooptic neuropathy (SMON)
Disulfiram	Chronic alcoholism	Sensorimotor peripheral neuropathy	Subacute or chronic visual loss	

Signs

1. Ophthalmoscopic findings include (Figure 5–24):
   - Early: hyperemia of the optic disc with blurred margins.
   - Later: pallor or cupping of the optic disc; thinning of the retinal arterioles.
2. Pupils: usually sluggish response to light, except in total loss of vision when the pupils are dilated and nonreactive.

Diagnosis

Serum methanol level are greater than 20 mg/dL.

Treatment

Ethanol should be given since it interferes with the metabolism of methanol. Treat the metabolic acidosis.

Prognosis:

Visual loss may be minimized with prompt treatment.

Ethambutol

General

1. This drug is used as an antituberculous agent.
2. The L form of ethambutol is primarily responsible for the toxic optic neuropathy, whereas the D form is responsible for the therapeutic effect.
3. Ocular toxicity is dose related, with an optic neuropathy most likely to occur at doses greater than 25mg/kg/day, although visual loss has been documented to occur at lower doses.
   - Onset: no earlier than 2 months after starting the medication. Median onset is 7 months.
   - Greater susceptibility for the development of optic neuropathy in patients with

renal tuberculosis as the drug is excreted via the kidneys.

Signs

1. Visual field: central scotoma, bitemporal or peripheral constriction.
2. Optic nerve: initially normal, followed by optic atrophy.

Prognosis

Vision usually improves slowly after the drug is discontinued, however, some patients may be left with permanent visual loss.

Tobacco (also known as tobacco-alcohol amblyopia)

The role of tobacco alone in producing optic neuropathy has not been clearly elucidated. It may be that patients with malnutrition are predisposed to developing tobacco optic neuropathy. Tobacco may impair the absorption of vitamin B_{12}. Some investigators suggest that the cyanide present in tobacco produces a cyanide optic neuropathy, although this has yet to be proven conclusively. The disease is found to be more common in pipe smokers.

TABLE 5–18. MEDICATIONS PRODUCING OPTIC NEUROPATHIES

Cisplatin
Isoniazid
Sulfonamides
Vincristine
Chloramphenicol
Disulfiram

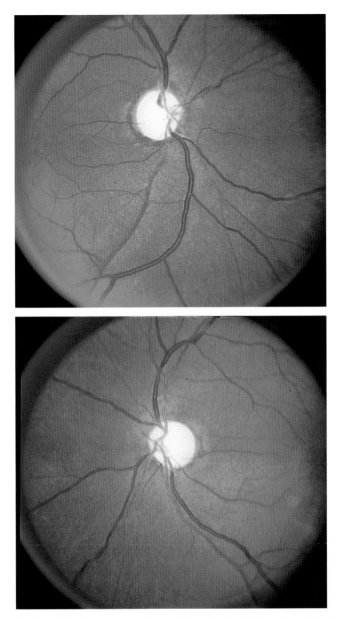

Figure 5–24. *Bilateral optic disc pallor in a patient who lost vision after drinking methanol.* (Courtesy of Neil R. Miller, MD.)

PAPILLEDEMA

Papilledema is defined as optic disc elevation, almost always bilateral, caused by increased intracranial pressure.

Epidemiology and Etiology

Any condition that produces increased intracranial pressure may produce papilledema.

Stages of Papilledema

There are several stages in the development of papilledema that occur over days or weeks depending on the cause.

1. *Insipient* (early) papilledema is characterized by mild disc hyperemia and minimal opacification of the peripapillary nerve fiber layer (Figure 5–25A). Spontaneous venous pulsations may be lost.
2. *Acute* (well-developed) papilledema shows unequivocal opacification of the nerve fiber layer with the presence of nerve fiber layer hemorrhages in the peripapillary area (Figure 5–25B).
3. *Chronic* papilledema is characterized by an optic disc that appears less hyperemic than in the earlier acute stages, and is less likely to have hemorrhages. There may be white concretions in the optic nerve (pseudodrusen), which are presumed accumulations of damned-up axoplasm due to the papilledema itself. Optociliary shunt vessels may begin to develop at this stage. Visual loss also begins to accelerate at this stage (Figure 5–25C).
4. *Atrophic* papilledema is the final stage of the disease. This is the process in which the optic nerves are pale, at times flat, and there is usually marked visual acuity and visual field loss (Figure 5–25D).

Clinical Characteristics

Symptoms

1. The patient may be completely asymptomatic.
2. Headaches may be present.
3. Transient visual obscurations lasting seconds and occurring mainly when the patient changes position or bends over and then stands up quickly are typical of papilledema.
4. Decreased vision occurs from optic nerve involvement when the papilledema is chronic. Acuity may be decreased because of fluid or folds in the macula (Figure 5–26) even in acute papilledema.
5. Diplopia due to unilateral or bilateral CN VI palsy.
6. Nausea and vomiting.

Signs

1. Optic disc changes:
   - Bilateral swollen hyperemic optic discs.
   - Blurring of disc margin and opacification of the retinal nerve fiber layer that produces obscuration of the peripapillary retinal blood vessels.
   - Papillary or peripapillary retinal hemorrhages.
   - Loss of venous pulsations.
   - Dilated tortuous retinal veins.
2. Visual field deficits begin with an enlarged blind spot and as the papilledema becomes chronic, progress to overall depression of the visual field, then the development of arcuate visual field defects, and only later the involvement of central fixation.
3. Visual acuity is lost late in the development of chronic papilledema. Acuity may be de-

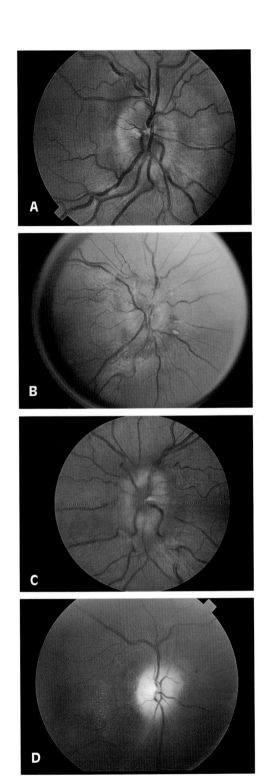

Figure 5–25.
A. Incipient papilledema.
B. Acute papilledema.
C. Chronic papilledema with horizontal folds radiating from the disc.
D. Atrophic papilledema.

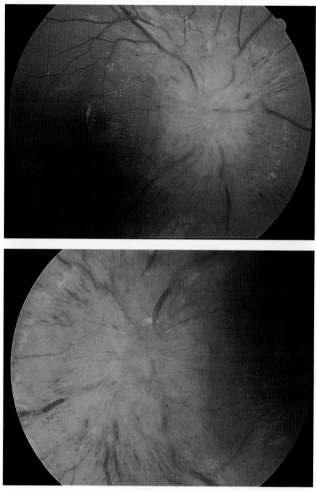

Figure 5–26. *Papilledema with fluid and exudates in the macula causing decreased acuity.*

pressed in acute papilledema when the swollen optic disc produces retinal folds, exudates or hemorrhages in the macula.

4. Unilateral or bilateral CN VI palsy.

Differential Diagnosis

Papilledema is not the only cause of an elevated optic disc. Inflammatory, ischemic or infiltrative processes may cause optic disc edema. Ophthalmoscopically, a congenitally elevated optic disc may be confused with papilledema, thus the term pseudopapilledema (see p. 95).

The most frequent causes of papilledema are listed in Table 5–19.

Investigations

All patients who are discovered to have any stage of papilledema constitute a medical emergency. They require immediate imaging to rule out an intracranial mass lesion or hydrocephalus. MRI is the best test to obtain, however, CT scanning is acceptable as an emergency procedure to rule out a mass lesion.

TABLE 5-19. FREQUENT CAUSES OF PAPILLEDEMA

Intracranial tumors: primary or metastatic
Pseudotumor cerebri
Sagittal sinus thrombosis
Aqueduct stenosis
Subdural or epidural hematoma
Arteriovenous malformation
Subarachnoid hemorrhage
Other: brain abscess, encephalitis, meningitis

Treatment

The treatment of the papilledema is directed primarily at the underlying cause. If this is not possible, treatment of the papilledema itself with a shunting procedure or optic nerve sheath fenestration to preserve vision may be considered.

PSEUDOTUMOR CEREBRI

Papilledema may develop in young women who are somewhat overweight. This condition is known as *pseudotumor cerebri* (PTC), or idiopathic intracranial hypertension (IIH). This disorder is not limited to young, overweight women, but may be seen in men or in thin patients of both genders. Usually, however, patients are overweight or have a history of recent weight gain.

The diagnostic criteria for PTC are:

1. Normal CT or MRI of the brain.
2. Increased CSF pressure on lumbar puncture with an otherwise normal CSF composition.
3. Absence of focal neurologic signs except CN VI palsies.

Etiology

There are two large categories of PTC.

1. The idiopathic variety of PTC, called by some IIH, but referred to by others as the

PTC syndrome. No identifiable cause for the papilledema is ever found in these patients.
2. Several conditions or agents may produce increased intracranial pressure including pregnancy, vitamin A, tetracycline, and corticosteroids. In addition, patients may have papilledema as a result of intracranial venous sinus thrombosis.

Clinical Characteristics

Symptoms

1. Headache is usually present but may be absent.
2. Transient visual obscurations.
3. Visual loss if chronic.
4. Double vision: due to CN VI palsies.
5. Tinnitus.
6. Dizziness.
7. Nausea and vomiting.

Signs

1. Bilateral optic disc edema.
2. Visual field deficits, which may be mild (enlarged blind spot) to severe. Nerve fiber bundle defects or depression of central acuity occurs with chronic papilledema.
3. Unilateral or bilateral CN VI palsy.

Investigations

1. Detailed history to identify any medications or toxins that may be producing this syndrome.
2. MRI to exclude an intracranial mass or hydrocephalus is performed in all patients, even if they fit the clinical profile of PTC (Figure 5-27).
3. Magnetic resonance venography (MRV) is the best test to rule out intracranial venous sinus thrombosis. We believe that MRV should be performed on all patients suspected of having PTC (Figure 5-28).
4. Lumbar puncture should be performed in all patients who do not have a mass lesion or hydrocephalus. This will document that

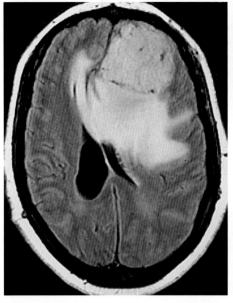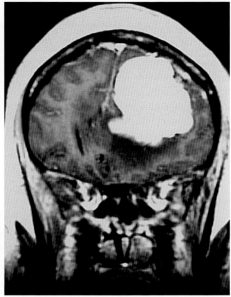

Figure 5–27. *Young, obese woman, with chronic papilledema, who on axial and coronal MRI was found to have a large meningioma and not pseudotumor cerebri as the cause of the papilledema.*

the cerebrospinal fluid pressure is elevated, but is otherwise normal in its formulation.

Treatment

1. In the event of an identifiable medicinal cause, for example, tetracycline or vitamin A ingestion, immediate discontinuation of the agent is indicated.
2. In intracranial venous sinus thrombosis, there is some debate about the treatment, but most authorities prefer aggressive anticoagulation. These patients should also be investigated for coagulopathies.
3. In PTC patients who are losing vision from the papilledema, the treatment options include:
   - Weight loss (approximately 10 to 15% of body weight in overweight patients) is effective.
   - Acetazolamide beginning at 1 g per day, and increasing as tolerated. There is no

firm evidence that any other diuretic is effective in the treatment of PTC.
- Optic nerve sheath fenestration if visual loss is profound at presentation or is progressing in the presence of chronic papilledema and headache is not a prominent symptom.
- Lumboperitoneal shunt is the procedure of choice if headache is severe.
- Repeat spinal taps should not be used as a routine treatment in PTC. There are only rare instances in which we believe they should be employed, for example, in a pregnant woman who is losing vision, in whom medication is inadvisable, and optic nerve sheath fenestration or shunting is contraindicated.
- Systemic corticosteroid administration is to be avoided except to lower intracranial pressure for a short period of time prior to surgical intervention for progressive visual loss.

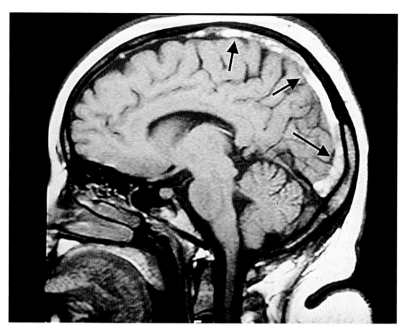

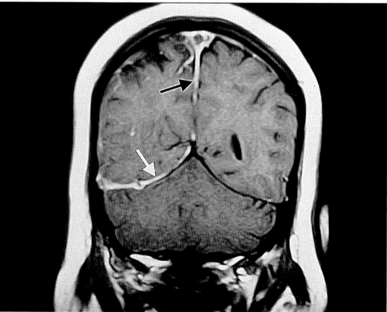

Figure 5–28. *Patient with papilledema shows increased signal due to thrombosis in the sagittal* (black arrow) *and transverse sinus* (white arrow).

OPTIC NERVE GLIOMA

This benign tumor of the optic nerve usually occurs in children and is often found in association with neurofibromatosis type 1 (NF-1).

Etiology and Epidemiology

These tumors are true neoplasms of the optic nerve and are most commonly juvenile pilocytic astrocytomas. They are commonly (30%) associated with NF-1. Optic nerve gliomas are the most common infiltrative tumor of the optic nerve.

Clinical Characteristics

Symptoms

1. Decreased vision: the majority of patients with optic nerve gliomas develop symptoms and signs within the first decade of life, and over 90% will present before the second decade.
2. Proptosis is the presenting characteristic if the bulk of the tumor is in the orbit. The proptosis is associated with features of an anterior optic neuropathy

Signs

1. A RAPD if asymmetric or unilateral.
2. Optic nerve-type visual field defects.
3. Proptosis that may be progressive.
4. Ocular motility disturbances: usually a sensory esotropia or exotropia.
5. Optic disc may show (Figure 5–29):
   • Swelling
   • Pallor: the most common optic disc finding
   • Optociliary shunt vessels: occasionally seen.
6. Associated signs and symptoms of NF-1 (Table 5–20).

Investigations

CT scan will reveal a circumscribed fusiform enlargement of the optic nerve (Figure 5–30). MRI scan of the optic nerve and the brain, however, is the diagnostic procedure of choice. It will characterize the tumor as being isolated or as part of a more extensive intracranial disease. The typical MRI characteristics of an optic glioma are (Figure 5–31):

1. Fusiform enlargement of optic nerve with or without associated enlargement of optic canal.
2. Hypointense or isointense on T1.
3. May show enhancement after injection of gadolinium, but the enhancement is not as pronounced as that produced by meningioma.
4. "Kinking" of optic nerve within orbit: seen exclusively in patients with NF-1.
5. Increased T2 signal around the nerve (pseudo CSF signal).

All patients diagnosed with an optic nerve glioma should be investigated for evidence of NF-1. Conversely, all patients diagnosed with NF-1 should be screened for the presence of optic nerve gliomas because 30% of gliomas occur in patients with NF-1.

Treatment

The treatment of optic nerve gliomas remains controversial.

Surgical resection may be considered if:

1. The glioma is extending intracranially but has not yet reached the optic chiasm.
2. There is severe proptosis causing corneal ulceration.

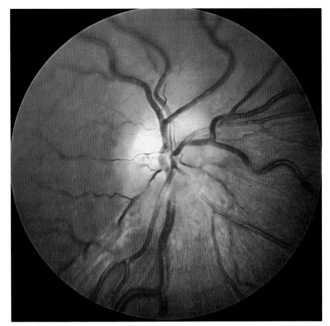

Figure 5–29. *The optic disc is elevated and hyperemic in the inferior two-thirds, with the superior one-third being paler. Optociliary shunt vessels are forming at the 9 o'clock position on the optic disc.*

3. No light perception vision at presentation is not universally accepted as an indication for surgical excision of the optic nerve.

If vision is poor or vision is progressively getting worse, treatment will depend on the patient's age.

1. Under 5 years of age, radiation therapy is not used, but chemotherapy may be administered. Chemotherapy may halt or retard growth of the tumor until the child reaches the age when radiation therapy may be administered safely.
2. Over 5 years of age, radiation to the optic glioma is the treatment of choice. However, it should be remembered that radiation therapy might produce side effects (Table 5–21).

Prognosis

The prognosis of isolated optic nerve gliomas is reasonably good for vision, with most patients maintaining stable visual acuity for years. Most optic nerve gliomas remain confined to one optic nerve. In our experience, it is rare for an isolated optic nerve glioma to spread to the optic chiasm or to the contralateral optic nerve. Patients with more extensive intracranial gliomas, particularly those involving the hypothalamus, have a more progressive disorder and the process may progress to blindness and/or death. If the glioma involves the optic tracts and chiasm, vision may deteriorate, but survival is usually not affected.

TABLE 5–20.   FEATURES OF NEUROFIBROMATOSIS TYPE 1

Cutaneous
  Café au lait spots: flat light brown patches
    Adults usually have more than six
    Appear during the first year of life and increase in size and number
  Axillary freckling: becomes obvious around the age of 10 years
  Fibroma mulluscum: predunculated flabby pigmented nodules that may be widely distributed
      throughout the body
  Plexiform neurofibroma: larger and less well defined than fibroma molluscum
Skeletal
  Congenital bone defects: aplasia of greater wing of sphenoid (may produce pulsating enophthalmos
      or exophthalmos)
  Acquired scoliosis
  Facial hemiatrophy
  Short stature
  Mild macrocephaly
Ocular features
  Eyelid and anterior segment
    Eyelid plexiform neuroma
    Prominent corneal nerves
    Lisch iris nodules: present in 95% of patients
    Congenital ectropion uveae
  Other
    Glaucoma: rare, but if present it is usually unilateral and congenital; approximately half will have
        ipsilateral facial hemiatrophy and upper eyelid neurofibroma
    Choroidal hamartoma
Other features
  Neural tumors: may develop in the brain, spinal cord, and the cranial, peripheral, and sympathetic
      nerves
  Malignancies
    Embryonal tumors of childhood or neurofibrosarcoma (5%)
    Pheochromocytoma
  Hypertension: secondary to renal artery stenosis or pheochromocytoma

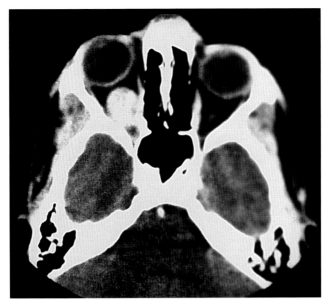

Figure 5–30. *CT scan of patient in Figure 5–29 shows fusiform enlargement of the optic nerve.*

TABLE 5–21. SIDE EFFECTS OF RADIOTHERAPY IN CHILDREN WITH OPTIC NERVE GLIOMA

Induction of secondary malignancies, endocrinopathies
Developmental delay
Vasculitis
Moya-moya disease
Radionecrosis of the temporal lobes
Leukoecephalopathy

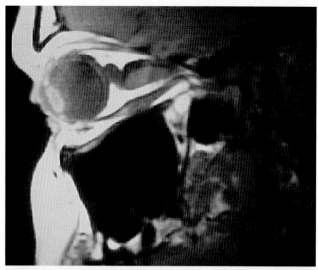

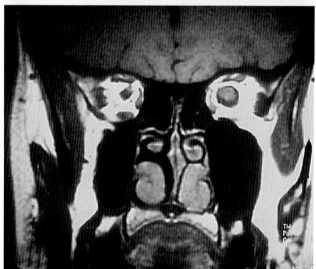

Figure 5–31. *Coronal and sagittal MRI of the left optic nerve glioma.*

MALIGNANT GLIOMA OF ADULTHOOD

This unusual tumor is a malignant glioma that involves the optic nerve. Malignant gliomas can be an isolated lesion or multicentric. This disorder usually affects older patients and is characterized by rapid progressive visual loss.

Etiology and Epidemiology

A malignant glioma of the brain.

Clinical Characteristics

Symptoms   Visual loss: in one or both eyes, that is rapidly progressive over a period of weeks or months.

Signs

1. Decreased vision that is progressive.
2. A RAPD if asymmetric or unilateral.
3. Optic nerve-type visual field deficits, which rapidly progress to no light perception vision.
4. Patients may present initially with a swollen optic disc and are often diagnosed as having AION, or with a normal fundus (diagnosed erroneously as PION). Subsequently, a central retinal vein occlusion often develops and frequently progresses to central retinal artery occlusion (Figure 5–32).

Investigations

MRI scan that shows an enhancing lesion. The lesions are characteristic of malignant glioma of the optic nerve (Figure 5–33) and possibly other parts of the brain if the lesion is multicentric.

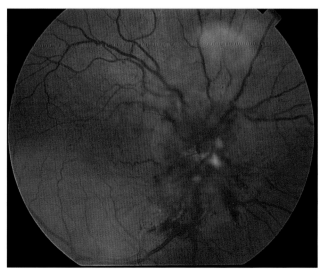

Figure 5–32.   *Patient with malignant glioma shows fundus picture of venous congestion, nerve fiber layer hemorrhages, and ischemia of the optic nerve head, consistent with combined retinal artery and vein occlusion.* (Courtesy of Robert C. Sergott, MD.)

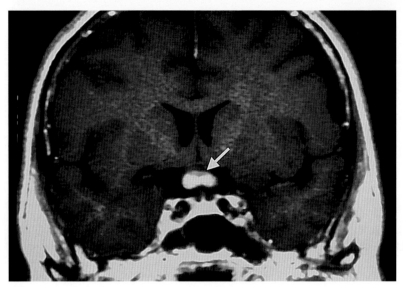

Figure 5–33. *Coronal MRI of patient with malignant glioma that has extended to the optic chiasm, which is enlarged and enhances* (arrow).

Treatment

Radiation therapy and chemotherapy are treatments that can be tried, however, the prognosis for vision and life is uniformly dismal. Most patients die within 1 year of diagnosis.

OPTIC NERVE SHEATH (PERIOPTIC) MENINGIOMA

Optic nerve sheath meningiomas are benign tumors that surround the optic nerve causing progressive visual loss.

Etiology and Epidemiology

Optic nerve sheath meningiomas are primary tumors that arise from meningoendothelial cells of the arachnoid. They usually involve the optic nerve in the orbit but may extend into the optic canal and through it to occupy the intracranial space. Meningiomas typically affect women over the age of 40 years and are a cause of progressive visual loss.

Clinical Characteristics

Symptoms Slow, progressive visual loss, which may be unilateral or bilateral, is the only symptom of this disorder. The tumors usually do not produce proptosis or ocular motility disturbances until very late in their course.

Signs

1. Decreased acuity.
2. Acquired dyschromatopsia.
3. Central visual field defects, central scotomas, or nerve fiber bundle defects.
4. A RAPD if asymmetric or unilateral.
5. The optic disc is usually swollen, with characteristic changes in the vasculature of the optic nerve head (optociliary shunt vessels) (Figure 5–34). As the tumor grows, the edema resolves and optic atrophy supervenes.

Investigations

CT scan shows the "tram-track" sign from calcifications along the optic nerve and tubular thickening of the nerve (Figure 5–35A). A meningioma usually appears as a thickened

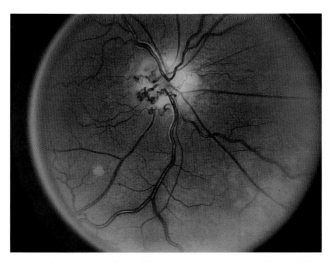

Figure 5–34. *Pale, elevated optic disc with optociliary shunt vessels in a blind eye. These are the typical findings of an optic nerve meningioma.*

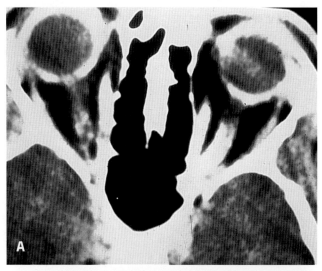
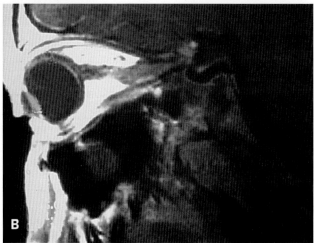

Figure 5–35. *A. Axial CT scan after contrast with typical appearance of bilateral optic nerve meningiomas.* *B. Sagittal MRI without contrast shows thickening of the optic nerve in the orbit and into the optic canal.*

optic nerve (Figure 5–35B) that enhances with gadolinium on MRI.

Treatment

Many patients may be observed without treatment if visual loss is not progressing. If vision is deteriorating, the preferred treatment is radiation therapy with conformal three-dimensional technology. There is no large series proving that this is the correct therapy, but there is compelling anecdotal information to support this therapy. There is no alternative therapy that appears to be effective. Surgery with attempted extirpation of the meningioma will result in blindness.

LEBER'S HEREDITARY OPTIC NEUROPATHY

Leber's hereditary optic neuropathy (LHON) is genetically inherited and is usually bilateral.

Etiology

Leber's hereditary optic neuropathy (LHON) is a disorder of mitochondrial (mt) DNA. There are several mutation sites in the (mt)DNA that are deemed to be primary mutations in that their presence alone can produce the disease. These sites are 11778, 3460, and 14484. It is estimated that approximately 90% of all the cases of LHON are due to one of these three mutations. A number of secondary mutations have also been identified.

Inheritance Pattern   All of the children of the mother will receive the trait, but only the female children are able to transmit the trait to the next generation. Both men and women can be afflicted with the optic neuropathy; however, the incidence is 9:1 men over women. The age of involvement is usually quite young, with most patients being involved in their teens or early twenties. It is unusual, but not unheard of, for patients to experience visual loss later in life.

Clinical Characteristics

Symptoms: Visual loss is the only ocular symptom of LHON. The visual loss is usually sequential, the second eye being affected within weeks to months of the first. Rarely, the eyes may be involved simultaneously or there will be only one eye involved.

Signs

1. Decreased visual acuity, usually 20/200 or worse. Vision may be lost abruptly or may progressively worsen over days.
2. RAPD if unilateral or asymmetric.
3. Dyschromatopsia.

4. Visual field defect, which is usually a central scotoma, with relative sparing of the peripheral vision.
5. Optic disc changes are characteristic of this disorder (Figure 5–36). The optic disc is usually swollen and hyperemic. There are often circumpapillary telangiectasias that are characteristic of LHON. The nerve fiber layer appears opacified, but there is no leakage from the optic disc on fluorescein angiography.

Differential Diagnosis

1. Optic neuritis: most patients are initially misdiagnosed as having optic neuritis because of the unilateral visual loss, swollen optic nerve, and very young age. Involvement of the second eye in a short period of time would be unusual for optic neuritis.
2. Ischemic optic neuropathy: this is an unusual finding in the age range that is usually affected by LHON.
3. Papilledema: this diagnosis is usually tendered when both optic nerves are swollen. However, the profound loss of vision in the presence of optic disc edema that is not chronic papilledema, establishes that this is not the correct diagnosis.

Investigations

1. Determination of genetic mutation. Laboratory testing is available for the primary and secondary mutations.
2. Fluorescein angiography is employed to demonstrate the peripapillary telangiectasias and the absence of leakage from the optic disc.

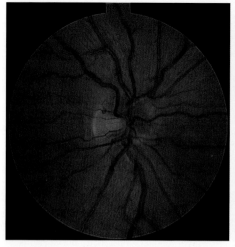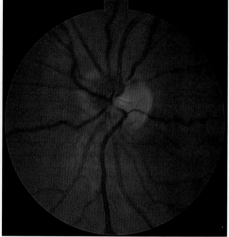

Figure 5–36. *Bilateral disc elevation. The right disc (left) is more hyperemic; the left (right) is developing pallor in the papillomacular area. The vision was lost first in the left eye.*

3. MRI scan may show subtle enhancement of the affected optic nerve, but neuroimaging is unnecessary in this disorder.

Associated Clinical Features

1. Cardiac conduction defects, usually preexcitation syndromes, are seen in some patients with LHON.
2. A MS-like disorder may appear in some patients.

Visual Prognosis

Usually the vision remains poor once LHON has occurred. Some patients, however, may experience recovery of visual acuity months to years later. This can occur by a gradual fading of the central scotoma or by the development of a small, clear area in the midst of the central scotoma, allowing the patient better visual acuity (Figure 5–37). Patients with the primary mutation 14484 tend to have the best chance of visual recovery, whereas those with the 11778 mutation have the poorest. Patients who are afflicted at a younger age appear to have a higher chance of visual recovery.

Treatment

No treatment is available for LHON.

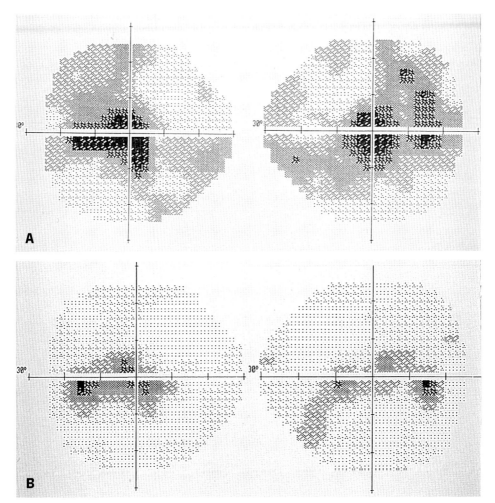

Figure 5–37. *A. Visual fields of a patient with Leber's hereditary optic neuropathy with dense central scotomas and vision of 20/400 bilaterally. B. Vision has improved to 20/25 OD and 20/40 OS, 2.5 years later. The central scotomas are much less dense bilaterally.*

DOMINANT OPTIC ATROPHY

Dominant optic atrophy (DOA) is statistically the most frequently inherited optic neuropathy.

Epidemiology/Etiology

The estimated prevalence of DOA is approximately 1:50,000. It is inherited in a dominant fashion. Genetic analysis has isolated one of the DOA genes (OPA1) on chromosome 3q28 to 29.

Clinical Characteristics

Symptoms

1. Decreased acuity usually occurs by age 10 years but may be minimal and go unnoticed by the patient for years.
2. Acquired dyschromatopsia, with many patients having tritanopia (blue/yellow) as the predominant color vision anomaly (Figure 5–38), as opposed to other optic neuropathies that have a deutanopia (red/green) type color defects. Some patients with DOA will have nonspecific color confusion.

Signs

1. The acuity loss is bilateral and progressive but does not usually fall below 20/200.
2. Bilateral central or cecocentral scotomas.
3. Pallor of the optic disc temporally affecting the papillomacular bundle area (Figure 5–39).

Differential Diagnosis:

Other bilateral optic neuropathies, mainly toxic or nutritional.

Investigations

A D-15 or Farnsworth-Munsell 100 Hue test may be used to document the tritanopia. Genetic testing is not available commercially.

Management

Genetic counseling. No therapy is effective.

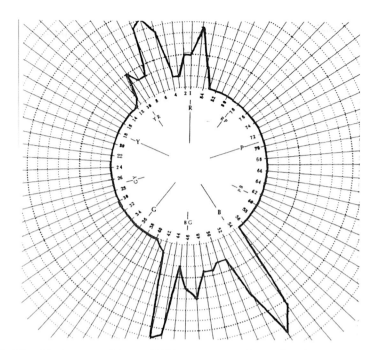

Figure 5–38. *The Farnsworth-Munsell 100 Hue axis is a blue-yellow deficiency, characteristic of DOA.*

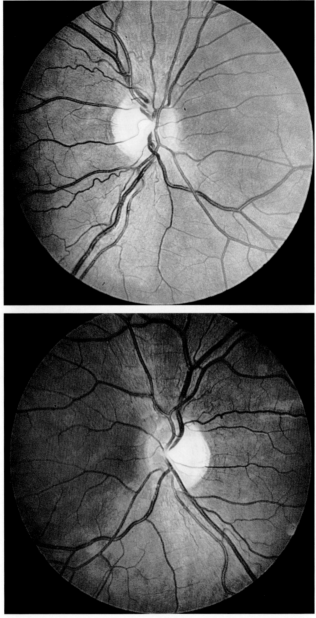

Figure 5–39. *There is sectoral pallor in both optic discs in the papillomacular bundle area characteristic of a DOA.*

CONGENITALLY ANOMALOUS DISCS (PSEUDOPAPILLEDEMA)

The normal optic disc is a rounded structure in the fundus and usually consists of a central cup. The disc is relatively flat to the retinal surface. Elevation of the optic disc above the retinal surface may be an acquired phenomenon (papillitis, papilledema), but also may be congenital. This condition may be bilateral and may be confused with papilledema due to increased intracranial pressure, thus the term "pseudopapilledema."

Etiology

This is a congenital phenomenon and tends to be familial.

Clinical Appearance

The characteristics of a typical congenitally anomalous optic disc (Figure 5–40) are as follows.

1. Is devoid of a physiologic cup.
2. Has the blood vessels originating at the center of the disc.
3. Is yellow or gray in color, not hyperemic.
4. Has abnormalities of the large blood vessels including loops, coils, and multiple branching patterns.
5. Some congenitally anomalous discs contain hyaline bodies (drusen) (Figure 5–41; see p. 97).
6. Normally the retinal nerve fiber layer is devoid of myelin. Occasionally myelin does extend from the retrolaminar optic nerve into the retina appearing as opacified white areas of nerve fibers (Figure 5–42). They may cause confusion with papilledema when they are in the immediate peripapillary area.

Differential Diagnosis

Congenitally anomalous discs may be confused with the acquired disc elevation of papilledema. Table 5–22 contrasts the appearance of a congenitally anomalous disc with that of true papilledema.

Investigations

If the ophthalmoscopic appearance is typical of a congenitally anomalous disc, and/or the presence of hyaline bodies or myelinated nerve fibers has been documented, no further investigations are required.

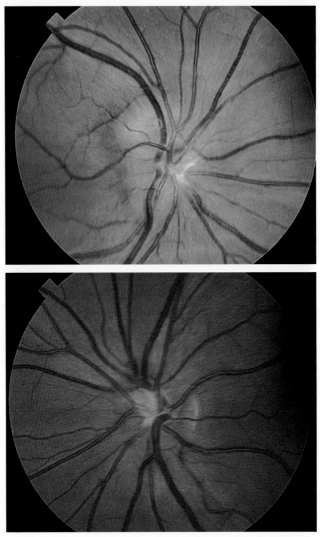

Figure 5-40. *Congenitally anomalous disc. Optic discs are elevated with no physiologic cup. There is a remnant of glial tissue centrally on each disc. The retinal nerve fiber layer is not opacified.*

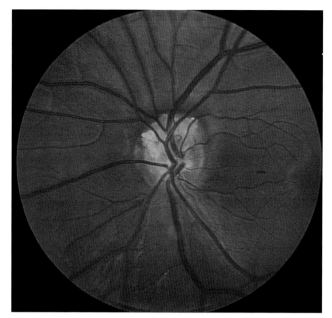

Figure 5–41. *Congenitally anomalous optic disc with visible drusen superiorly. Note absence of retinal nerve fiber layer striations superiorly and their presence inferiorly, where there are no drusen.*

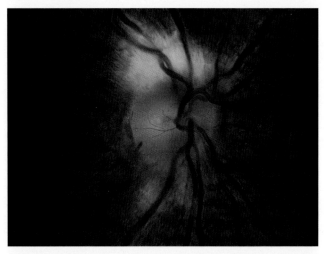

Figure 5–42. *Myelin appears as white areas at the poles of the disc. Nerve fiber layer striations are seen inferiorly and at the edges of the superior area of myelin.*

TABLE 5–22.

	Congenitally Anomalous Disc	Papilledema
Laterality	Unilateral in one-third of patients	Bilateral
Disc color	Yellowish white	Hyperemic
Vessels	Anomalous large vessels with loops, coils, and multiple branching patterns	Increased capillaries on the disc surface
Cup	Absent	Present until late in the course
Hemorrhage	Unusual	Frequent
Other	Drusen (hyaline bodies) may be visible in the disc	Small concretions (pseudodrusen) are a sign of chronic disc edema
Retinal nerve fiber layer	Clear	Opacified

OPTIC DISC DRUSEN

These are accumulations of a *hyaline* material within the optic nerve. The drusen become progressively larger as the patient ages.

Epidemiology and Etiology

Inherited: the exact pattern is not known, although it has been suggested to be an irregular dominant trait with incomplete penetrance. Drusen tend to occur almost exclusively in Caucasians and are present in about 1% of the population. They are bilateral in approximately 70% of cases.

Symptoms

Usually the patient is asymptomatic. The disorder is usually detected on a routine ophthalmologic examination. However, occasionally, the associated visual field defects may be symptomatic.

Signs

1. Acuity is usually intact.
2. A RAPD if unilateral or asymmetric.
3. Visual field defects are usually arcuate defects, especially inferiorly. They can slowly progress. It is rare, however, for central acuity to be decreased by drusen of the optic disc.
4. Characteristic appearance of glistening material within the optic disc (Figure 5–43). In children, drusen usually remain "buried" in small, pink optic disc and become apparent in the second decade. These discs have indistinct margins and anomalous branching of the central retinal vessels may occur (see congenitally anomalous disc).
5. Several types of hemorrhage may be associated with disc drusen:
   - Peripapillary nerve fiber layer (splinter) hemorrhages.

- Hemorrhages on the optic disc overlying the drusen.
- Peripapillary, crescent-shaped hemorrhages that may be subretinal or beneath the retinal pigment epithelium (RPE). The typical alterations of the peripapillary RPE occur on resolution of these subRPE hemorrhages.
- Vitreous hemorrhage.
- Bleeding from a subretinal neovascular membrane that may be adjacent to or distant from the optic disc (Figure 5–44).
- Peripapillary hemorrhage from AION that can occur on the background of drusen.

Differential Diagnosis

Papilledema if bilateral and the optic disc drusen are buried within the substance of the disc and not visible ophthalmoscopically.

Investigations

1. Visualization of the drusen ophthalmoscopically establishes the diagnosis and no further testing is necessary.
2. If the drusen are not obvious, B-scan ultrasonography will establish their presence (Figure 5–45).
3. CT scan may also detect the presence of optic disc drusen (Figure 5–46).
4. Drusen will autofluoresce before the injection of dye during fluorescein angiography (Figure 5–47).

Management and Therapy

No therapy is effective.

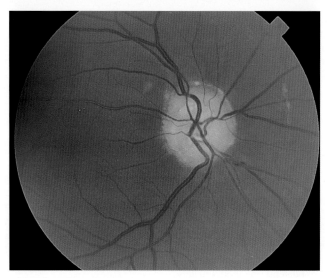

Figure 5–43. *The optic disc contains drusen, which are best seen at the 7 and 10 o'clock positions on the optic disc.*

Special Comment

If the patient has elevated intraocular pressures, it is often impossible to tell if the progressive visual field loss is due to drusen or glaucoma because in glaucoma, disks with drusen often do not develop typical cupping.

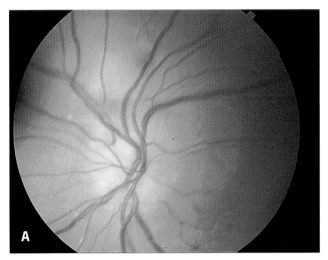

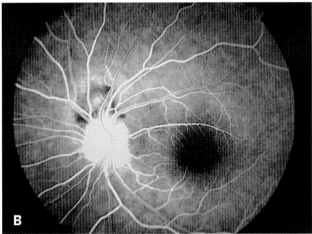

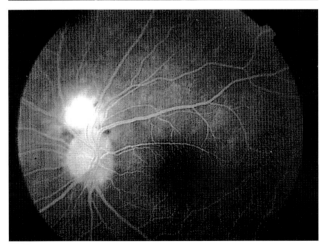

Figure 5–44. *A. Congenitally anomalous disc with visible drusen. There is a crescent-shaped hemorrhage at the superior pole with retinal nerve fiber layer edema.* *B. Flourescein angiography shows early blockage of background fluorescence by the hemorrhage and edema at 12 o'clock (0.21.8 sec). Leakage of dye with late straining is typical of a subretinal neovascular membrane.*

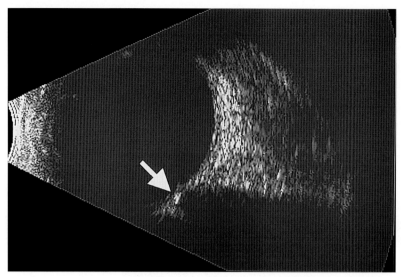

Figure 5–45. *Ultrasonogram in B-scan mode illustrating calcified disc drusen* (arrow).

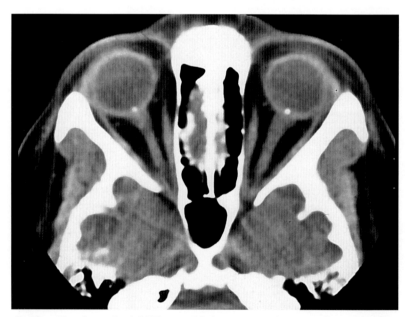

Figure 5–46. *Unenhanced axial CT scan with drusen appearing as a white spot in the area of each optic disc.*

CHAPTER 5   OPTIC NERVE DISORDERS

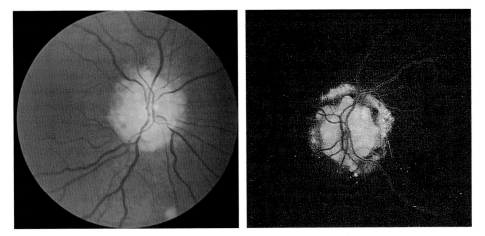

Figure 5–47. *Optic disc drusen (left) showing autofluorescence (right).*

OPTIC NERVE HYPOPLASIA

Optic nerve hypoplasia is a congenital anomaly in which the optic nerve is smaller than usual. This phenomenon is present from birth, and does not progress. It is frequently associated with other CNS abnormalities. Complete absence of the optic disc (aplasia) is very rarely encountered.

Etiology and Epidemiology

Several risk factors are associated with the development of optic nerve hypoplasia. These include a young maternal age and maternal insulin dependent diabetes mellitus. Also, the use of alcohol (fetal alcohol syndrome) and various drugs (illicit drugs, quinine, and some anticonvulsants) during pregnancy have been implicated as causes of optic nerve hypoplasia.

Clinical Characteristics

Symptoms

1. Decreased vision in one or both eyes.
2. Vision may vary from normal acuity with a constricted visual field to no light perception.
3. Patients may experience growth retardation and hormonal imbalances.

Signs

1. RAPD if unilateral or asymmetric.
2. Strabismus is often present.
3. The optic disc is smaller than normal and often surrounded by a ring of choroid (double ring sign) (Figure 5–48). Histopathologically, the outer ring corresponds to the normal junction between the lamina cribrosa and the sclera. The inner ring represents the termination of retina and retinal pigment epithelium over the lamina cribrosa.
4. Astigmatism is frequently associated with hypoplasia.

Investigations

1. The primary investigation in patients with optic nerve hypoplasia is endocrinologic. These patients will often have growth retardation and corticotropin deficiency; therefore, they should be referred to a pediatric endocrinologist.
2. MRI scanning might be considered given that the optic nerve hypoplasia may be associated with intracranial developmental abnormalities which include:
   - hemispheric migration anomalies (schizencephaly, cortical heterotopia),
   - intrauterine or perinatal injury (periventricular leukomalacia, encephalomalacia, porencephaly), and
   - posterior pituitary ectopia.

Treatment

The only treatment is occlusion therapy to combat any amblyopia that might have developed as a result of the optic nerve hypoplasia and/or strabismus.

Special Forms

Hemihypoplasia: Topless Disc Syndrome A special form of optic nerve hypoplasia occurs in children of insulin dependent diabetic mothers. This form is characterized by hypoplasia of the superior portion of one or both optic nerves (Figure 5–49A) and rather dense inferior arcuate or altitudinal visual field defects (Figure 5–49B) Often, the patients are unaware of these visual field defects since they exist from birth.

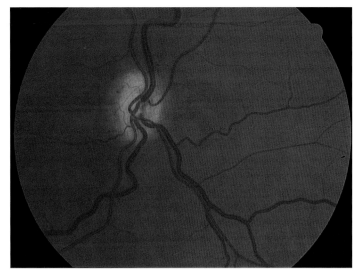

Figure 5–48. *There is almost no disc tissue. The central white area is sclera. Note that the retinal nerve fiber layer is absent and the retinal blood vessels are of normal size.*

Septooptic Dysplasia: de Morsier's Syndrome Septooptic dysplasia refers to:

1. Small anterior visual pathways
2. Agenesis of corpus callosum
3. Absence of septum pellucidum

4. Other associated features may include:
   - Pituitary dwarfism
   - Diabetes insipidus

This may not be as specific a syndrome as previously believed.

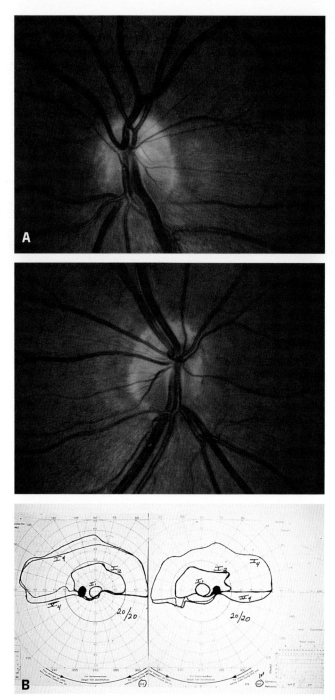

Figure 5–49. *A. The optic discs are hypoplastic superiorly. The central vessels, which are of normal caliber, exit at the very top (not the center) of the disc.* *B. Kinetic perimetry shows bilateral inferior altitudinal defects with preserved central acuity.*

CHAPTER 5 OPTIC NERVE DISORDERS

OPTIC DISC COLOBOMAS

Colobomas of the optic disc are congenital anomalies in which the optic disc is dysplastic and may be larger than normal, or has other defects that are visible ophthalmoscopically.

Etiology and Epidemiology

Colobomas are the result of the failure of fusion of the embryonic fissure during the fifth to sixth weeks of gestation. They are usually isolated findings and are rarely associated with intracranial disorders, such as transphenoidal encephaloceles and other signs of a midline cleft syndrome. Commonly, they occur bilaterally.

Clinical Characteristics

Symptoms Decreased vision to a variable extent in one or both eyes or the patients may be asymptomatic.

Signs

1. A RAPD if unilateral or asymmetric.
2. Optic nerve-type visual field defects that are not progressive.
3. Usually, they are positioned interiorly and can affect the optic disc, retina, choroid, inferior iris, and lens.
4. Common ophthalmoscopic findings (Figure 5–50):

- Enlarged disc that may be partially or completely excavated.
- Peripapillary pigmentary changes are common (either hyper- or hypopigmentation)
- The coloboma has a glistening white appearance.
- The retinal blood vessels are normal.
5. Serous retinal detachments: nonrheg-matogenous.
6. A variety of ocular anomalies may be associated with colobomas (Table 5–23).

Investigations

An MRI scan is not required since transsphenoidal encephaloceles are rarely encountered with colobomas but more frequently with the so-called morning glory disc anomaly (Figure 5–51).

Treatment

No treatment is effective, except for occlusion therapy for amblyopia that may have developed as a result of these dysplastic lesions of the optic disc.

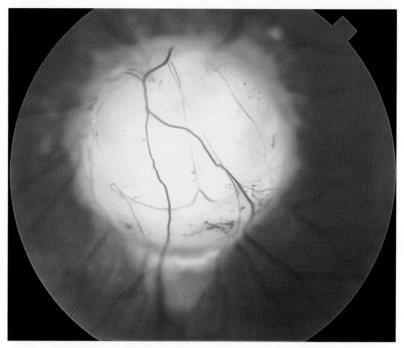

Figure 5–50. *The optic disc is enlarged, but there is disc tissue superiorly. There is minimal RPE pigmentation change and the defect extends inferiorly in the area of the embryonic fissure. The retinal vasculature is normal.*

TABLE 5–23. ASSOCIATED OCULAR FEATURES OF COLOBOMAS

Posterior lenticonus
Congenital optic disc pit
Hyaloid artery remnant
Posterior embryotoxin
Myopia
Strabismus (in children)

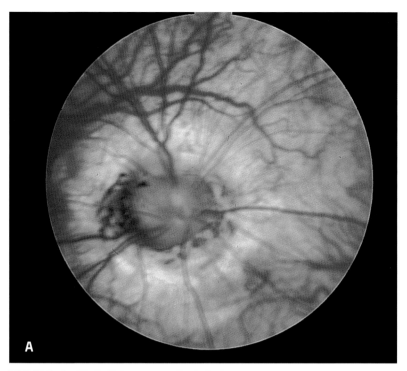

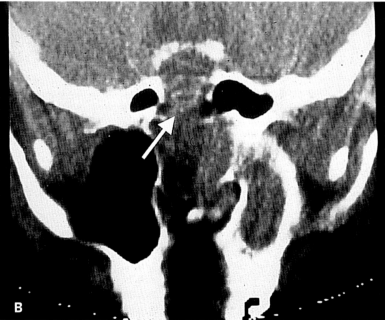

Figure 5–51.   *A. Morning glory optic disc in a patient with midline defects of the lip and palate.*   *B. Coronal CT scan shows midline defect in the sphenoid bone with herniation of tissue into the nasopharynx* (arrow).

OPTIC PIT

Optic pits appear as dark depressions in the optic nerve. They are typically located inferotemporally on the optic disc. They may communicate with the subarachnoid space.

Etiology and Epidemiology

The optic pit is a form of optic disc dysplasia that is thought to occur during development prior to the differentiation of the neural retina and the optic nerve head. It is actually a defect in the lamina cribrosa into which grow areas of dysplastic retina. The exact cause for the pit formation is unknown.

Clinical Features

1. Unilateral in 85%.
2. Round or oval depression that may be pigmented in a normal size optic disc (Figure 5–52).
   - Vary in size: $\frac{1}{4}$ to $\frac{1}{2}$ disc diameter.
   - Rarely, more than one pit may be present (Figure 5–53).
3. Located most frequently in the inferior temporal region of the disc.
4. Does not affect the disc margin (unlike coloboma) and the physiologic optic cup remains distinct.
5. Peripapillary chorioretinal atrophy with changes in the pigment epithelium where the pit is situated.
6. Abnormal vascular pattern:
   - Cilioretinal artery can be identified arising from the periphery of the pit.
   - Retinal vessels cross the optic pit
7. Retinal elevation: develops in 30% of cases and may cause: (Figure 5–54) visual field defects and metamorphopsia.

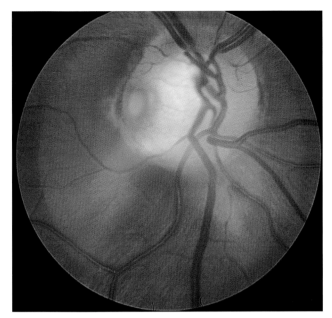

Figure 5–52. *Optic pit of right disc in the typical location. Note pigmentation of pit and adjacent chorioretinal and retinal pigment epithelium defects.*

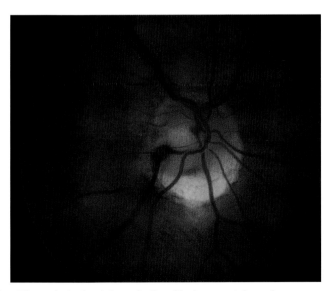

Figure 5–53. *Three pits in the right optic disc. The largest pit has a large artery and vein. The smaller pits are at 6 and 10 o'clock.*

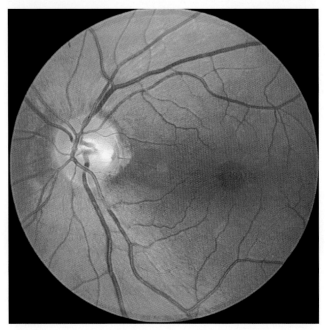

Figure 5–54. *Optic pit of the left eye with apparent cilioretinal artery. Macula edema is the cause of decreased vision.*

TRAUMATIC OPTIC NEUROPATHY

Traumatic optic neuropathy (TON) occurs by a variety of mechanisms in the setting of closed head trauma.

Epidemiology and Etiology

Traumatic optic neuropathy occurs most frequently in young men, the population that is most frequently involved in both penetrating and nonpenetrating trauma.

Mechanisms by which traumatic optic neuropathy may be produced include:

1. The most frequent cause of traumatic optic neuropathy is *blunt head trauma* producing an acceleration-deceleration injury. The patient's head is moving rapidly forward and strikes a firm object, rapidly decelerating. This action causes a shearing force that separates the meningeal blood supply of the optic nerve from the optic nerve itself.
2. Patients may develop a traumatic optic neuropathy from *compression* by a bony fragment as a result of fracture of the optic canal (Figure 5–55), or from a hematoma that is developing in a closed tight compartment, for example, the optic canal or the orbital apex. Orbital compartment syndrome is an ophthalmic emergency that necessitates immediate management.
3. *Penetrating injury* is a less frequent cause of direct TON due to the relative laxity of the intraorbital optic nerve, which allows for absorption of the impact of the penetrating object. In addition, because the dural tissue of the optic nerve sheath is thick, it resists laceration. If penetration of the dura of the optic nerve does occur, then TON can present by several mechanisms, including transection of nerve fibers or compression from hemorrhage, edema, or impingement on the nerve by a foreign body (Figure 5–56). This final mechanism must be considered if the foreign body is localized at the orbital apex, where the optic nerve is inflexible due to tethering by the annulus of Zinn.

4. Complete or partial *avulsion* of the optic nerve can occur, usually from a direct blow to the eye. In most cases, prepapillary vitreous hemorrhage occurs relatively quickly, obscuring the view of the optic nerve head and making definitive diagnosis difficult.
5. A rare cause of direct TON is *optic nerve sheath hematoma*. This typically presents with signs of progressive visual loss and optic neuropathy, and necessitates the presence of venous congestion or occlusion on funduscopic examination. Arterial compromise may also be noted. CT imaging may show expansion of the optic nerve sheath, but this finding may also be seen in cases of intraconal orbital hemorrhage, where blood within the fat compartment around the optic nerve sheath may give the false impression of a true nerve sheath hematoma.

Clinical Characteristics

Symptoms

1. The primary symptom of traumatic optic neuropathy is visual loss. The visual loss may be total or partial.
2. Visual field defects may be plotted when some vision is preserved.

The tempo of loss of vision is important in determining its cause. The shearing force injury of traumatic optic neuropathy results in immediate visual loss. The compressive traumatic optic neuropathy from bony fracture or hematoma develops more slowly, with the patient initially having preserved vision, but then losing vision over a period of hours. Avulsions result in sudden visual loss.

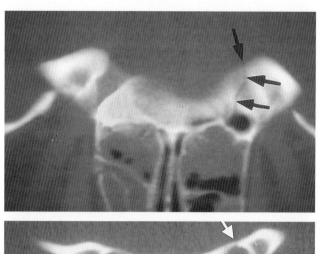

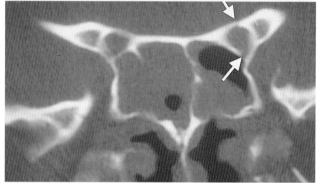

Figure 5–55. *Fracture of the optic canal shown in axial* (black arrows) *and coronal* (white arrows) *views.*

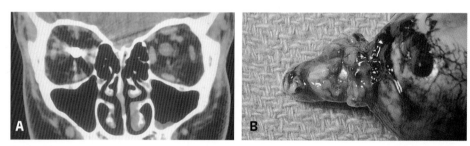

Figure 5–56. *Immediate visual loss from a perforating globe injury by a BB pellet.* **A.** *Coronal CT shows proximity of the BB to the optic nerve.* **B.** *Enucleation specimen demonstrates the BB lodged in the optic nerve.*

Signs

1. Decreased visual acuity.
2. Impaired color vision.
3. A RAPD if it is a unilateral optic neuropathy.
4. Orbital hemorrhage presents as severe ecchymosis and lid edema. Proptosis and external ophthalmoplegia are usually present (Figure 5–57). The orbit will be tight to palpation and lid opening may require the use of retractors. Intraocular pressure may be elevated and signs of vascular compromise may be seen on funduscopic examination.
5. Ophthalmoscopy may reveal a partial or complete avulsion of the optic nerve with a ring of hemorrhages at the site of injury.

Investigations

In blunt head trauma, the patient should undergo a CT scan first, with special views of the optic canal, to detect any impinging fractures (Figure 5–58). If no metallic foreign bodies are seen, an MRI may be considered to look for hematomas that might be causing compression. These two tests are most important to perform in a situation where the patient had preserved or relatively preserved vision after the trauma, and then begins to lose vision. If one of these two causes is identified, decompression of the optic nerve by removal of the compressive cause should be done expeditiously.

A case can be made for no investigation in a patient who suffers immediate loss of vision with head trauma, since this is most likely due to shearing force injury.

Treatment

A traumatic optic neuropathy study was attempted, but failed to enroll an adequate number of patients to determine if high-dose intravenous corticosteroids have a beneficial effect on this condition. Most clinicians will treat patients with high-dose corticosteroids if these medications are not otherwise contraindicated.

There have been reports of optic canal decompression even in patients with normal CT scans, resulting in improvement of vision. These results are controversial and most neuroophthalmologists and oculoplastic surgeons in the United States do not employ this method of treatment.

Orbital compartment syndrome from orbital hemorrhage is treated effectively with inferior cantholysis (Figure 5–59). Lateral canthotomy alone is ineffective therapy. Cantholysis should be performed expeditiously in cases of optic neuropathy to maximize the potential for visual recovery.

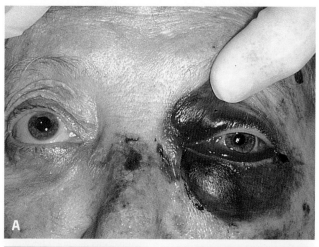
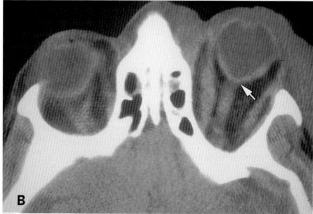

Figure 5–57. *Orbital hemorrhage with optic neuropathy.* **A.** *Note the ecchymotic, tense eyelids along with proptosis and external ophthalmoplegia.* **B.** *Axial CT reveals a "tenting sign" of the globe: distortion of the eyeball by a combination of proptosis and tethering by the optic nerve* (arrow).

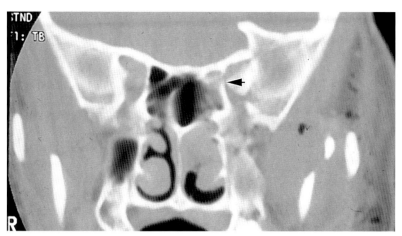

Figure 5–58. *A lateral will fracture is displaced medially and compresses the optic nerve between it and the medial orbital wall* (arrow) *at the orbital apex.*

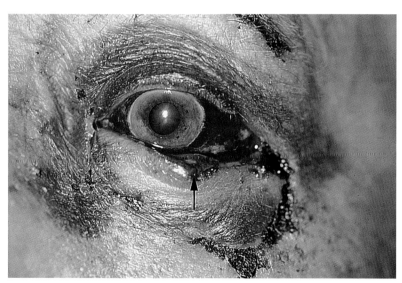

Figure 5–59. *Orbital hemorrhage with successful inferior cantholysis. Note the marked medial migration of the lateral canthus* (arrow). *When performed expeditiously, visual recovery is often dramatic.*

Chapter 6

OPTIC CHIASM

As they extend intracranially, the optic nerves, rise and move medially to come together to form the optic chiasm. This structure, which is the confluence of the optic nerves, sits approximately 10 mm above the dorsum sellae. Disorders of the optic chiasm initially may present with visual acuity loss. The clinical demonstration of a chiasmal pattern of visual loss enables the physician to order the appropriate tests and to establish the correct diagnosis. The single most important test in determining if the optic chiasm is the involved site producing visual loss is the visual field. The confluence of the optic nerves and the crossing of the nasal fibers at the chiasm, combined with the 90-degree rotation that the visual fibers undergo en route to the chiasm from the retina, orients the nerve fibers along the vertical meridian. Therefore, visual field defects at the optic chiasm and posteriorly will characteristically respect the vertical meridian on perimetric testing.

Types of Visual Field Abnormalities in Chiasmal Disease

1. Junction scotoma: classically, this is a combination of a central scotoma in one eye and a temporal hemianopic defect in the other (Figure 6–1). The localization of this visual field defect is the junction of the optic nerve, on the side of the central scotoma, and the optic chiasm. The classically accepted cause for this pattern of visual loss is the existence of Willbrand's knee, which is the anterior extension of the nasal crossing fibers from one eye into the opposite optic nerve. A lesion of the right optic nerve will produce a central scotoma on the right, and because of involvement of the inferior nasal

fibers from the left eye, a superior temporal defect in that left eye. Recently, there has been some controversy as to whether Willbrand's knee is an anatomic or just a functional entity. Modern studies in monkeys have failed to show the anatomic existence of Willbrand's knee; however there is general agreement that the junctional scotoma still is a valid sign that localizes lesions to the junction of the optic nerve and chiasm.

A lesion may involve only the crossing visual fibers at the anterior angle of the optic chiasm. This produces a monocular temporal hemianopic defect with no visual field loss in the contralateral eye (Figure 6–2).

2. Bitemporal hemianopia: the classic visual field abnormality produced by lesions of the body of the optic chiasm. The visual field defects may be complete (Figure 6–3A) or incomplete (Figure 6–3B), but they always obey the vertical meridian. In most cases, however, pure bitemporal hemianopic defects are infrequent. Usually, there is decreased acuity in one or both eyes.

3. Homonymous hemianopia: a parasellar lesion may produce an incongruous homonymous hemianopia by involving the optic tracts. This may occur with masses that are directed posteriorly or because the optic chiasm is prefixed. The homonymous hemianopia often is associated with a central scotoma and a RAPD on the side of the mass lesion. This is known as the *optic tract syndrome* (see the following discussion).

Any patient with decreased vision of unknown etiology requires a visual field examination. When the visual field shows one of the defects associated with chiasmal involvement, the next test to perform is an MRI scan.

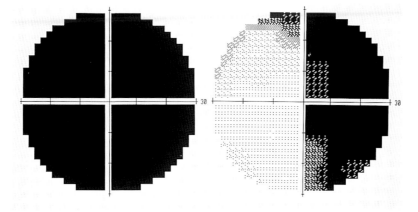

Figure 6–1. *Patient with neurosarcoidosis has a dense central scotoma in the left eye and a temporal hemianopic defect on the right.*

Etiology

Approximately 90% of the disorders that produce chiasmal lesions are mass lesions. The most frequent of these are listed in Table 6–1.

Clinical Characteristics of Chiasmal Disease

Symptoms

1. Visual loss is the most frequent and most important symptom of parachiasmal disor-

ders, other symptoms may be associated with it but are infrequent in the absence of visual loss.

2. Headache may be seen with pituitary tumors and implies a stretching of the meninges in the area.

3. Diplopia: parachiasmal lesions may cause double vision in several ways:
   - Extension into the cavernous sinus: since the most frequent cause of a chiasmal syndrome is a mass lesion, it may extend laterally into the cavernous sinus to involve CN III, IV, or VI on one or both sides. This produces a variety of diplopia

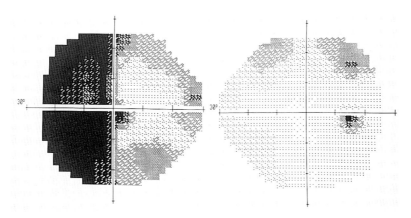

Figure 6–2. *Patient with a large suprasellar meningioma presented with a temporal hemianopic defect and decreased vision in the left eye with no defect in the right.*

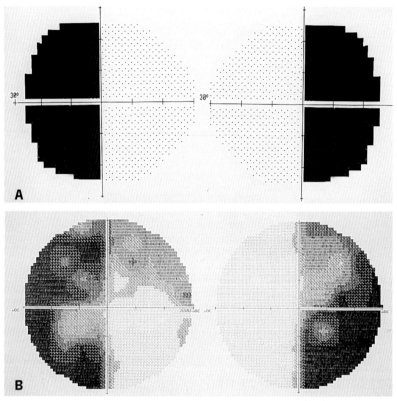

Figure 6–3. *A. Complete bitemporal hemianopia.* ***B.*** *Incomplete bitemporal hemianopia.*

patterns depending on which cranial nerves are affected (Figure 6–4).

- A form of diplopia without presumed ocular misalignment is the so-called *hemifield slide phenomenon*. This phenomenon

TABLE 6–1. FREQUENCY OF PITUITARY MASS LESIONS*

Type	Percentage
Pituitary Adenoma	50–55%
Craniopharyngioma	20–25%
Meningioma	10%
Glioma	7%

*Other causes of chiasmal syndrome such as aneurysm and other compressive lesions are relatively uncommon.

occurs when patients lose the ability to fuse because the bitemporal hemianopia produces a situation where there is no binocular area of overlapping or interlocking visual field. Thus, the eyes can slide in a vertical plane. These patients have difficulty adding a column of numbers because the numbers from one line suddenly appear on the line above or below.

4. Post-fixation blindness: this is a peculiar type of visual disability that afflicts patients with chiasmal disease. The bitemporal hemianopia causes patients to have an area of blindness immediately beyond the point of fixation when viewing something at near (Figure 6–5). This occurs because when converging on a point, the area beyond the

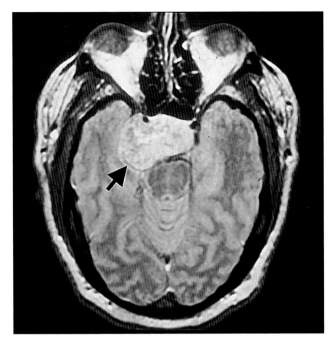

Figure 6–4. *Axial MRI shows large pituitary tumor extending into the cavernous sinus* (arrow). *The patient presented with a pupil involving CN III palsy.*

point of regard falls within the blind bitemporal fields.

Signs

1. Decreased acuity is usually present, although a bitemporal hemianopia or other visual field defect may be present with normal acuity.
2. Acquired dyschromatopsia in one or both eyes.
3. Visual field defect (see previous discussion).
4. A RAPD is usually present with asymmetric or unilateral visual loss.
5. The optic disc may be normal or pale. Disc edema, or papilledema, is unusual, but may be seen especially with craniopharyngiomas.
6. Ocular misalignment is usually the result of involvement of the cranial nerves (III, IV, VI) in the cavernous sinus.
7. Endocrinologic signs and symptoms are often seen with chiasmal disorders and in-

clude pituitary insufficiency, amenorrhea galactorrhea syndrome, acromegaly, precocious puberty, diabetes insipidus, etc.

Specific Causes of Chiasmal Syndrome

Pituitary Tumors Pituitary tumors are the most frequent cause of the chiasmal syndrome. They may be endocrinologically inactive or may secrete a variety of hormones, which produce symptoms other than those produced by compression of the optic chiasm.

1. Tumors that secrete prolactin will produce an amenorrhea galactorrhea syndrome in women, and impotence in men.
2. Acromegaly occurs when tumors produce an excessive amount of growth hormone.

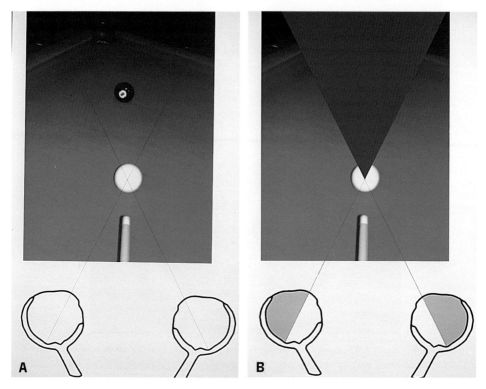

Figure 6–5. *Post fixational blindness.* **A.** *The normal view.* **B.** *The bitemporal hemianopia causes the area in front of the cue ball to disappear.*

3. Nelson's syndrome is characterized by acquired cutaneous hyperpigmentation and increased ACTH levels following a total adrenolectomy for Cushing's disease.

The diagnosis of the various forms of pituitary tumors is made by a combination of imaging and endocrinologic findings. The typical MR finding is one of a large mass lesion that displaces and distorts the optic chiasm. Because of its location 10-mm above the dorsum sellae, small pituitary tumors never produce visual field deficits. Tumors must extend out of the sella tursica and become quite large before they produce disturbances of visual acuity or visual field. This makes these tumors readily diagnosable by neuro-imaging (Figure 6–6A).

Several types of pituitary tumors are important to identify:

1. Prolactin-secreting tumors produce high levels of prolactin and because of this, are amenable to medical treatment. Prolactin-secreting pituitary tumors that produce visual loss usually produce prolactin levels over 1000 ng/mL (normal < 100 ng/mL). These tumors may dramatically decrease in size with dopamine agonist therapy. The visual field defects may disappear within weeks of instituting bromocriptine or cabergoline (see Figure 6–6).

2. Endocrinologically inactive pituitary tumors are the most frequent pituitary tumors and produce endocrine abnormalities such as hypothyroidism and hypopituitarism. These tumors are not amenable to medical treatment. In order to decompress the visual pathway, surgery and/or radiation is required.

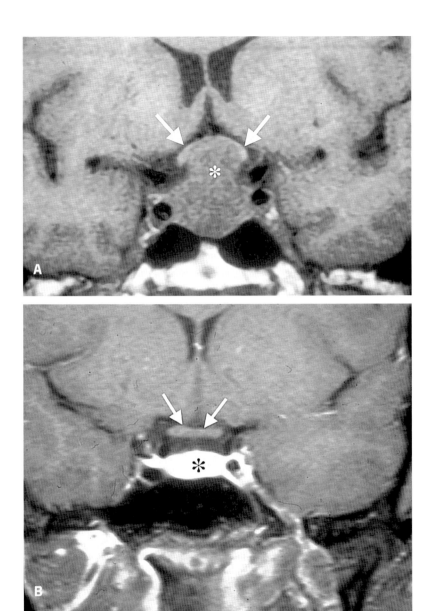

Figure 6-6. *A. Coronal MRI scan (left) showing a large prolactin secreting pituitary tumor (∗) capped by a distorted optic chiasm* (arrows). *B. Following the administration of bromocriptine, the pituitary tumor shrunk and the optic chiasm is in its normal position* (arrows) *without compression.*

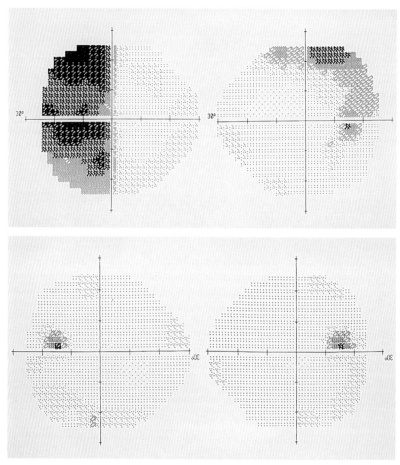

Figure 6–6. (*continued*) *Visual fields pre* (top), *and post* (bottom) *bromocriptine therapy show disappearance of the bitemporal hemianopia.*

3. Pituitary apoplexy is a special manifestation of pituitary tumors. While pituitary tumors produce slowly progressive, almost insidious visual loss, pituitary apoplexy is a dramatic event. The patient experiences *headache* (often as bad as the headache experienced in subarachnoid hemorrhage) and may suddenly develop *blindness* and/or *ophthalmoplegia* in one or both eyes. Pituitary apoplexy is due to a rapid expansion of a preexisting pituitary tumor because of swelling produced by hemorrhage into the tumor, which increases its size (Figure 6–7). This is an emergency. Patients often are suffering from hypopituitarism and hypocorti-solism and must be treated medically to restore their normal hormonal levels before invasive procedures are performed.

The role of the ophthalmologist following any treatment for pituitary tumor is to perform sequential visual fields, to go along with sequential MRIs, to document as early as possible any recurrence of these tumors.

A typical schedule for follow-up perimetry is:

- Every 3 months for the first year, then annually for 5 years.
- After 5 years, every 2 years.

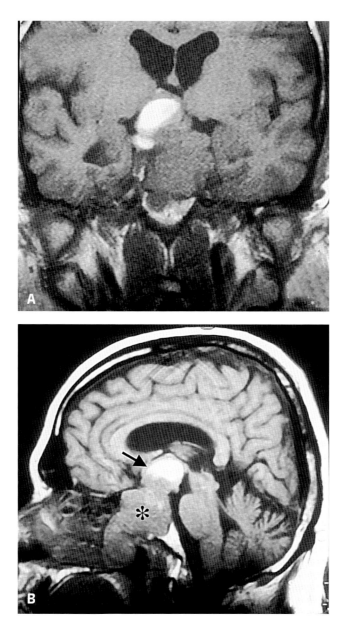

Figure 6–7. *Coronal and sagittal MRI of a large pituitary tumor (*) capped by a crescent of hyperintense blood* (arrow), *which caused rapid expansion of the tumor.*

Craniopharyngioma Craniopharyngiomas arise from Rathke's pouch, which is located between the anterior and posterior lobes of the pituitary gland. They are seen in children as well as adults. They may be solid or cystic, with the cysts filled with a viscous fluid that contains cholesterol-like flecks.

The signs and symptoms of craniopharyngioma include the following.

1. Visual acuity loss in one or both eyes.
2. Visual field abnormalities (see previous discussion).

3. Papilledema may be present, but is not common.
4. Endocrinologic abnormalities may occur.
5. Adults may become demented or confused.

DIAGNOSIS The diagnosis of craniopharyngioma is based on the visual field evaluation, indicating a chiasmal localization and the MR that is characteristic (Figure 6–8).

TREATMENT The treatment for craniopharyngioma is surgery. Most often, the tumor

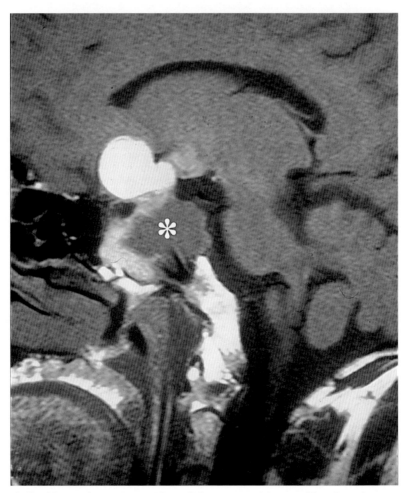

Figure 6–8. *Craniopharyngioma with a solid component (∗) capped by a hyperintense cyst filled with colloid material.*

cannot be removed in toto, therefore, postoperative radiation or chemotherapy to the tumor bed may be indicated. Close follow-up with visual fields and MRI scan is required because of the propensity of the craniopharyngioma to regrow.

Meningioma Parachiasmal meningiomas may be suprasellar or located in the area of the tuberculum sellae or planum sphenoidale (Figure 6–9). They are also slow growing tumors that often produce visual loss as the only sign. Endocrine abnormalities are much less likely to occur in meningiomas than in pituitary adenomas or craniopharyngiomas.

The treatment for parachiasmal meningiomas is surgery. Overaggressive surgical removal is to be discouraged, since this will often result in further loss of vision.

The ophthalmologist's role is to perform visual fields in the postoperative period.

Glioma Optic gliomas are intrinsic lesions of the optic chiasm that are relatively uncommon. They also produce a chiasmal syndrome with visual acuity and visual field loss, and are most frequently associated with neurofibromatosis. Approximately one-third of patients with neurofibromatosis type I (NF1) will have gliomas of the anterior visual pathways on MRI (Fig. 6–10).

The symptoms of chiasmal glioma are again those of visual loss and chiasmal visual field abnormalities (see previous discussion). The association of NF1 must raise the real possibility that the chiasmal syndrome is due to glioma.

A form of glioma may involve the optic chiasm in adults. This more aggressive glioma is known as malignant glioma of adulthood and is actually a glioblastoma of the anterior visual pathways. It progresses rapidly, and patients usually expire within 1 year (see Chapter XX).

The treatment of gliomas is controversial. Some clinicians recommend radiation therapy; chemotherapy is used in some patients, especially children under 5 years of age, where radiation therapy may produce long-term mental deficits.

Other Mass Lesions Any mass lesion in and around the optic chiasm may produce the same spectrum of clinical signs and symptoms. These include aneurysm, dermoid tumors, and metastatic lesions. The exact diagnosis is arrived at through neuroimaging and, at times, biopsy.

Follow-up of Parachiasmal Tumors

During the follow-up of treated parachiasmal tumors, the visual field may deteriorate. The causes are:

1. Regrowth of tumor.
2. Radiation necrosis of the optic chiasm if radiation has been administered (Figure 6–11).
3. Chiasmal prolapse into an empty sella (Figure 6–12).
4. Arachnoiditis is a rare cause of visual loss following surgery.

Non-Mass Lesions Causing Chiasmal Syndrome

Inflammatory lesions [lymphoid hypopysitis, demyelinating disease (Figure 6–13), sarcoidosis, etc] may produce a chiasmal syndrome with typical visual field and acuity loss. Thus, the responsibility of the ophthalmologist in evaluating a patient with unexplained visual loss is:

1. Perform a visual field.
2. If the visual field indicates a lesion that potentially involves the optic chiasm, perform a MRI scan.
3. If the MRI scan identifies a lesion involving the optic chiasm (tumors or nontumors), the patient should be referred to a neurologist or a neurosurgeon.
4. Following the treatment of chiasmal disorders (especially tumors), the role of the ophthalmologist is to perform sequential visual field testing to document any possible recurrence of the mass lesion.

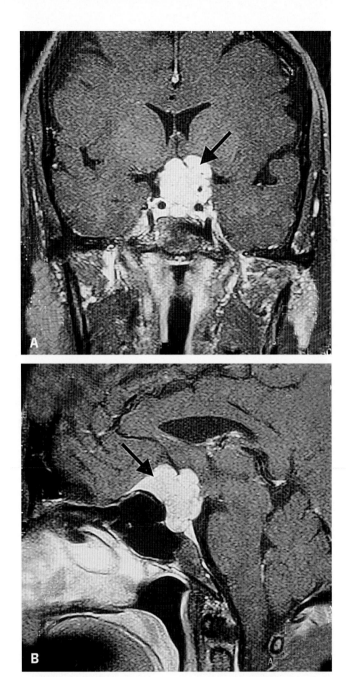

Figure 6–9. *Coronal and sagittal MRI showing parasellar meningioma* (arrow). *The patient's visual fields are seen in Figure 6–2.*

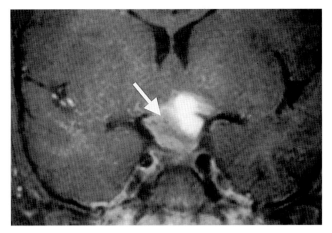

Figure 6–10. *Coronal MRI reveals a thickened optic chiasm* (arrow) *with enhancement of the glioma.*

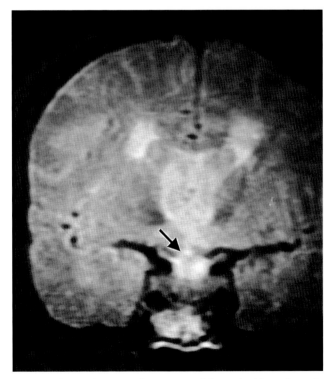

Figure 6–11. *Coronal MRI showing enhancement of the optic chiasm* (arrow) *consistent with radiation necrosis.*

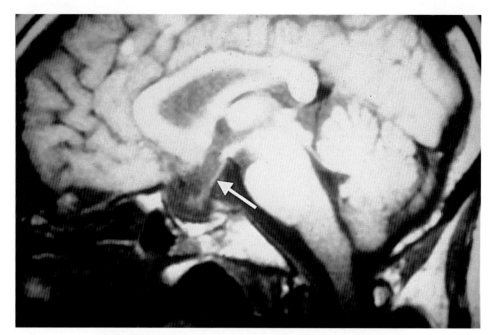

Figure 6–12. *Sagittal MRI with prolapse of optic chiasm* (arrow) *into an enlarged sella turcica following pituitary apoplexy.*

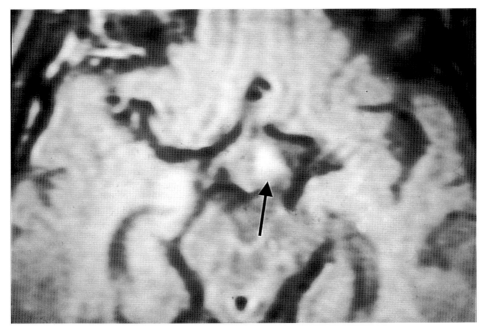

Figure 6–13. *Axial MRI showing demyelinating plaque* (arrow) *in the optic chiasm.*

Chapter 7

RETROCHIASMAL DISORDERS

The predominant visual sign of any lesion involving the post-chiasmal visual pathway is the *homonymous hemianopia.*

The form of the homonymous hemianopia will differ depending on what portion of the retrochiasmal visual pathway is involved.

1. Optic tract: this portion of the visual system is immediately behind the optic chiasm. Lesions in this area may produce one of two syndromes.

   Optic tract syndrome type I is the combination of ipsilateral decreased acuity, an incongruous homonymous hemianopia, and an ipsilateral RAPD (Figure 7–1). It is caused by large-mass lesions that involve the optic tract, optic chiasm, or even the optic nerve. The decreased visual acuity is due to the involvement of the optic nerve. The most frequent lesion that causes this form of the optic tract syndrome is the craniopharyngioma.

   Optic tract syndrome type II involves intrinsic lesions of the optic tract, usually produced by demyelinating disease or infarction. Visual acuity is intact, the RAPD is on the side opposite the lesion, and the homonymous hemianopia is complete or nearly so.

   Other findings associated with optic tract lesions are:
   - Optic disc changes: bow-tie atrophy on the side contralateral to the side of lesion (side with temporal field loss) and temporal pallor on the ipsilateral side.
   - Wernicke's hemianopic pupil: projecting light onto the retinal elements that subserve the "blind" hemifield produces a reduced or no pupillary response, but a normal pupillary response is elicited from testing the retinal elements that subserves the normal hemifield. Clinically, this phenomenon is difficult to produce.

2. Temporal lobe: lesions of the temporal lobe produce a homonymous hemianopia denser superiorly (Figure 7–2). The most frequent causes are tumors or following temporal lobectomy for seizures.

   Nonvisual manifestations of lesions of the temporal lobe include:
   - Headache
   - Auditory hallucinations or illusions
   - Disturbance of language (if dominant temporal lobe involved)
   - Disturbance of memory
   - Seizures manifested as transient changes in mood, emotions, and behavior
   - Uncinate fits: aura of unusual taste or smell followed by abnormal motor activity of the mouth and lips
   - A sensation of déjà vu

3. Parietal lobe: lesions of the parietal lobe produce a homonymous hemianopia that is denser inferiorly.

   Associated neuroophthalmic features may include:
   - Conjugate movement of the eyes to the side opposite the lesion on forced lid closure.
   - Abnormal optokinetic response when targets are moved to the side of the lesion.
     Neurologic features are:
   - Neglect of contralateral space, inattention (nondominant parietal lobe).
   - Impairment of complex sensory integration.
   - Gerstmann's syndrome: a lesion in the dominant parietal lobe may result in con-

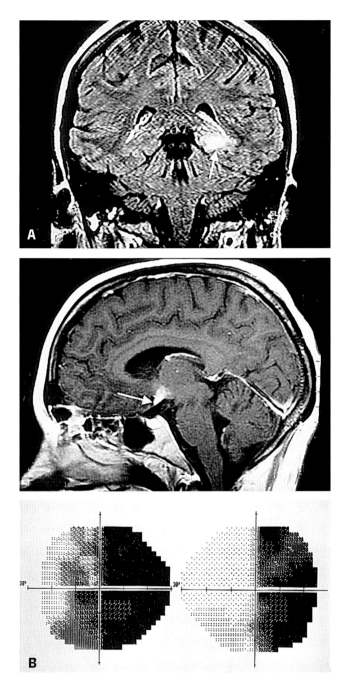

Figure 7–1. *A. Coronal and sagittal MRI scans show enhancement of the area of the left optic tract* (arrows) *in a patient with neurosarcoidosis.* ***B.*** *Visual fields show a right homonymous hemianopia with involvement of central fixation causing decreased visual acuity in the left eye.*

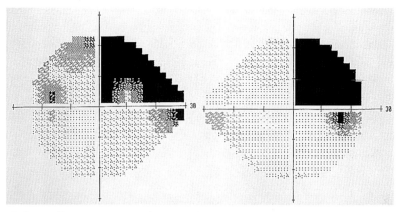

Figure 7-2. *Following temporal lobectomy, the patient had a right superior homonymous quandrantanopia characteristic of a temporal lobe lesion.*

tralateral homonymous hemianopia, finger agnosia, right-left confusion, agraphia, and alcalculia.

4. Occipital lobe: patients with occipital lobe visual field defects are most likely to seek care first from the ophthalmologist because their only symptom or sign is visual. These patients will often complain of difficulty reading and are frequently the recipients of multiple pairs of reading glasses before it is recognized that their difficulty is due to inability to see the next letter or word because of a right homonymous hemianopia or the inability to find the next line due to a left homonymous hemianopia.

As the visual fibers course toward the occipital lobe, they become more segregated and, therefore, visual field defects due to posterior lesions are more congruous. Incomplete homonymous hemianopias of occipital origin are, therefore, exquisitely congruous. Visual field deficits caused by lesions anterior to the occipital lobe do not produce this degree of congruity.

There are several hallmarks of occipital lobe visual field defects. These are:

a) *Temporal crescent sparing or involvement:* the temporal crescent area lies anteriorly in the visual cortex. It represents a portion of nasal retina from one eye that has no shared associated (temporal retinal) fibers. Therefore, it is the one

place in the visual radiations where a lesion may produce a unilateral visual field defect. The field defect is crescent shaped and its widest extent is in the horizontal meridian where it extends from 60 degrees to 90 degrees. It is worth remembering that the most used automated static perimetry programs will fail to detect this abnormality because it is further in the peripheral field than these tests measure. The most frequent type of visual field defect associated with this area is sparing of this temporal crescent. The homonymous hemianopia will appear incongruous because there is a rim of preserved vision capping the outer most portion of the temporal visual field defect. MRI scan shows a lesion sparing the anterior portion of the occipital cortex (Figure 7-3). Rarely is this area involved in a manner to produce loss of the crescent alone.

b) *Macular sparing:* a homonymous hemianopia of occipital origin may split fixation or may skirt around fixation by about 2 to 3 degrees (macular sparing) (Figure 7-4). This is true sparing and is seen only with occipital lobe lesions. Macular splitting may be seen with homonymous hemianopias from any area of the visual radiations.

c) *Paracentral homonymous scotomas:* lesions of the tip of the occipital lobe pro-

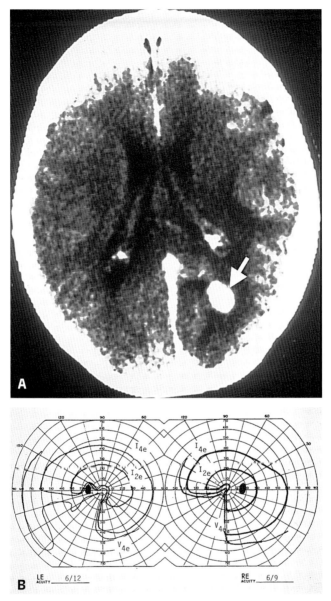

Figure 7–3. *A. Axial CT scan of a patient with a metastatic lesion to right occipital lobe. B. Perimetry shows left inferior quandrantanopia with temporal crescent sparing in the temporal portion of the left visual field.*

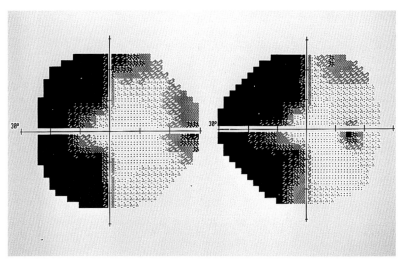

Figure 7-4. *A left homonymous hemianopia with macular sparing in a patient with an occipital lobe lesion.*

duce homonymous scotomas that are exquisitely congruous.

d) *Bilateral occipital lobe disease:* various patterns of visual field loss can be seen with bilateral occipital lobe disease. These include:

- Bilateral homonymous scotomas: may look like bilateral central scotomas.
- "Ring" scotoma: a small island of central vision remains as a result of bilateral, congruous homonymous scotomas with macular sparing.
- Bilateral altitudinal field defects (usually inferior): lesions that actually produce bilateral homonymous quadrantic defects.
- "Checkerboard" field defect (Figure 7–5): crossed quandrantanopia. This is caused by lesions, usually consecutive events, which affect the superior occipital lobe above the calcarine fissure on one side and the inferior occipital lobe below the calcarine fissure on the other side.

The other characteristics of occipital lobe disease that are important to the ophthalmologist include:

a) Cortical blindness: bilateral occipital lobe disease can produce blindness. These patients are often diagnosed initially as malingerers or hysterics because they complain of very poor or no vision, yet their pupils react briskly and their fundus is normal. At times, the patient will deny the blindness and fabricate a visual environment (Anton's syndrome). In any patient with these signs and symptoms, bilateral lesions of the occipital lobe must be ruled out by MRI. The most frequent cause of cortical blindness is stroke in the older age group, although it may be seen after arteriography and in the peripartum period associated with pregnancy induced hypertension. Cortical blindness may also be seen following chiropractic manipulation of the neck, carbon monoxide

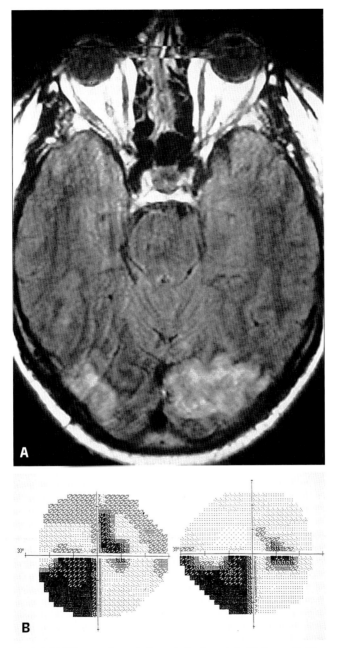

Figure 7–5. *A. Axial MRI scan shows infarcts in both occipital lobes. B. There are bilateral relatively congruous visual field defects that correspond to the occipital lobe lesions.*

poisoning, cyclosporin A toxicity, and occipital lobe seizures.

b) Dyschromatopsia: acquired dyschromatopsia is usually an anterior visual pathway phenomenon (optic nerve or chiasm). There is a form of acquired dyschromatopsia (cerebral dyschromatopsia) that is produced by *bilateral* occipital lobe lesions.

c) Palanopsia: this phenomenon consists of a persistent or recurrent visual image after the stimulus has been removed. This is typical of an occipital lesion and is usually associated with a homonymous hemianopia. It may be produced, however, by the ingestion of hallucinogens, specifically LSD.

d) Hallucinations: occipital lobe hallucinations are not rare. They are unformed as opposed to formed hallucinations produced by lesions of the temporal lobe.

In summary, any patient who has a homonymous hemianopia, be it complete or incomplete, congruous or incongruous, requires an MRI scan as the next test.

MIGRAINE

Migraine is the most frequent cause of homonymous visual field loss. The hemianopia is transient but infrequently may become permanent.

Epidemiology

Migraine is a very frequent phenomenon that can present in various forms. The exact prevalence of migraine is difficult to calculate because of different classifications and descriptions of headaches.

Classification

The International Headache Society classification of migraine is as follows.

1. Migraine without aura
2. Migraine with aura
3. Ophthalmoplegic migraine
4. Retinal migraine
5. Childhood periodic syndromes that may be precursors to or associated with migraine
6. Complications of migraine
7. Migrainous disorder not fulfilling above criteria

Patients with migraine with aura will often consult the ophthalmologist first.

Clinical Characteristics

Symptoms

1. The patient may experience a *prodrome* with a sense of uneasiness, drowsiness, or depression.
2. The *aura* of migraine varies, but the typical visual aura is that of a positive (although it may be negative) scotoma with jagged, often shimmering edges. The scotoma usually expands in size and tends to move across the visual field. The aura is usually in the form of jagged lines—the classic fortification scotoma (Figure 7–6), but it also may be bright lights. The aura typically lasts for 20 to 30 minutes and may be followed by a headache, or the end of the aura may terminate the attack (acephalgic migraine).
3. The *headache* phase of migraine with aura occurs immediately after the aura, but if the aura is particularly long, there may be some overlap and the headache may begin while the aura is still present. It is distinctly unusual, but possible, for the aura to occur after the headache. The quality of the headache varies from severe and incapacitating to relatively minor. It may last for hours.

Signs

1. Between attacks, the patient has a normal examination.
2. If examined during the attack, the patient may have a homonymous hemianopia if the origin of the migraine is cortical.

Differential Diagnosis

1. Vitreous traction is usually distinguishable from migraine because photopsias produced by vitreous traction last seconds to only a few minutes, whereas the visual aspect of migraine lasts much longer.
2. Occipital lobe lesions.
3. Arteriovenous malformations (AVM) (Figure 7–7) usually cause the most concern as being migraine mimickers. The visual phenomenon of AVMs is usually more short lived than those of migraine and may occur after the headache has already begun.

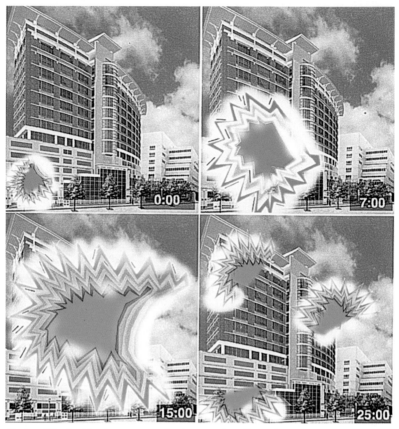

Figure 7–6. *The fortification scotoma begins peripherally and gradually involves the entire visual field. It usually clears without producing a permanent defect.*

Investigation

We do not routinely image patients who present with typical migraine:

1. Onset before age 50, although migraine may occur de novo after that.
2. Family history of migraine or migraine equivalents as a child.
3. Classical description of the aura and/or headache, which lasts the appropriate length of time.
4. The visual aura alternates sides.
5. There is no fixed neurologic or ocular deficit following the migraine.

However, patients who present with the following characteristics receive further investigation.

1. The visual aura is inevitably in the same location in visible space.
2. The headache precedes the visual aura. Although this is sometimes seen in migraine, it is uncommon and suspicious for an AVM.
3. A fixed neurologic (including visual) deficit is noted following termination of the event.
4. Any other circumstance that would render the episode atypical for migraine.

MRI is the first test to do in any patient who is going to be evaluated for atypical migraine.

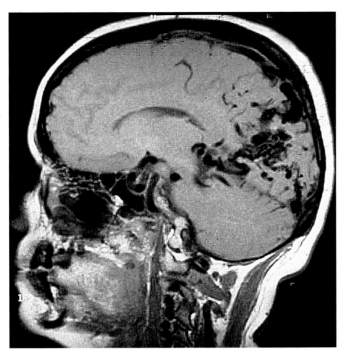

Figure 7–7. *Sagittal MRI showing a large arteriovenous malformation that mimicked migraine.*

Treatment

Treatment of migraine involves a variety of factors, including:

1. Elimination of precipitators, for example foods (wine, cheese, chocolate), stress modification.

2. If behavior modification does not prevent migraine, a series of medications are available that may be used at the appearance of the aura to prevent the headache phase, during the headache phase to shorten it, and prophylactically in the inter-headache phase to prevent migraines from recurring.

Chapter 8

NONPHYSIOLOGIC VISUAL LOSS

Patients may present with complaints that mimic organic disease but are factitious. The most frequently encountered forms of these disorders involve the afferent visual system and consist of:

1. No vision (one or both eyes)
2. Decreased vision (one or both eyes)
3. Visual field loss (one or both eyes)

No Vision

No vision is often the easiest to detect. The examiner has to prove that vision exists in the purported blind eye(s). This can be accomplished by one of several methods.

1. Mobility testing: watch patient enter room and perform manual tasks. Patients with nonphysiologic visual loss often claim to be unable to perform any tasks of mobility.
2. Functional tests: a blind person will be able to sign his or her name without difficulty. A patient with feigned visual loss may claim to have difficulty doing this.
3. Outstretch arm-to-nose test: a blind person will be able to easily touch their nose after the arm has been extended; whereas a person with feigned visual loss, not realizing this is a proprioceptive and not a visual test, may miss his or her nose completely.
4. Threat: a sudden threatening movement toward the patient's face that causes him or her to react appropriately proves the existence of vision.
5. Mirror test: hold a mirror up to the blind eye(s) and ask the patient to concentrate on

focusing straight ahead. Then, tilt the mirror horizontally and vertically. The more the patient tries to steady the eye, the more it will move in concert with the mirror tilt.
6. Optokinetic response: the development of an optokinetic response to an appropriate target in a blind eye is evidence of preserved vision.
7. Relative afferent papillary defect. In the setting of one blind and one normal eye, a RAPD (or amaurotic pupil) must be demonstrated. Absence of the RAPD is proof that the problem is factitious. This is not necessarily true with bilateral blindness since patients who are blind from bilateral occipital lobe disease have normally reacting pupils.

Decreased Vision

Patients with factitious incomplete visual loss are often more difficult to diagnose. The examiner must (by any means available) have the patient read better than his claimed defect. The technique must be tailored to the patient and to whether the patient is claiming unilateral or bilateral decreased vision. Techniques include:

1. Encouragement: start at 20/10 line and slowly proceed up chart.
2. Fogging: confusing the patient so he reads with the "bad" eye when he believes he is reading with the "good" one. Add plus spheres in front of one eye so that the patient is actually being tested with the eye in which poor vision is claimed.

3. Retest VA at half the distance from the chart. The VA should be twice as good.
4. Near vision: with appropriate add, this should be equivalent to distance vision.
5. Worth four-dot test: If all four dots are seen, vision is better than hand-motions.
6. Stereopsis: patients with 60 seconds of arc must have 20/20 in one eye and at least 20/40 in the other.
7. A series of devices, including stereoscopic and red-green projectors can be used to confuse the patient so that he reads with the "bad" eye when he believes he is reading with the "good" one. All methods are legitimate tactics.

Visual Field Loss

Feigned visual field loss may be claimed either with preserved or decreased acuity. Formal perimetry, either automated-static or kinetic, will produce typical patterns of factitious visual field loss (Figure 8–1).

Examination of the patient with confrontation techniques or using a tangent screen and varying the distance between the patient and the target will often uncover the dissembler. As the distance from the patient increases, the normal visual field expands. Constriction (funnel vision) or nonexpansion (tunnel vision) of the visual field under these conditions is a nonphysiologic response. Remember that when the distance from the test surface is doubled, the size of the test object must also be doubled.

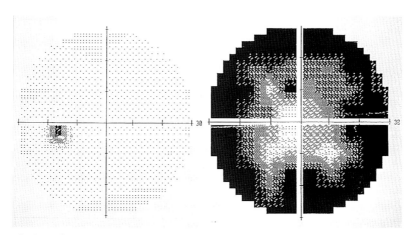

Figure 8–1. *The patient complained of poor vision in the right eye, but the right visual field showed a "clover-leaf" pattern consistent with nonphysiologic visual loss. The left visual field was normal and there was no RAPD.*

Chapter 9

NEUROOPHTHALMOLOGIC EXAMINATION— EFFERENT SYSTEM

Disorders of the efferent visual system result in either ocular misalignment or abnormalities in ocular motility without ocular misalignment. The most frequent symptom that prompts a neuroophthalmologic examination of the efferent system is **diplopia**. Other symptoms such as head tilts, face turns, etc., also require that evaluation of the efferent system be performed looking for disorders of ocular motility that do not produce diplopia.

The patient who presents with the symptom of diplopia should be approached in a systematic way to most efficiently identify the cause of diplopia and whether the diplopia has a potentially neuroophthalmic cause. There are several steps to follow to arrive at the correct diagnosis:

1. Identify **monocular diplopia.** The most important initial aspect of the diplopia evaluation is for the examiner to understand if the double vision is present only with both eyes open or is appreciated monocularly. Monocular diplopia is almost invariably due to an ocular disorder and is very rarely a manifestation of neuroophthalmologic disease. Patients with monocular diplopia therefore need not be subjected to intensive neurologic and neuro-radiologic investigations. If the patient has not cross-covered his eyes and does not know if the double vision persists when either eye is occluded, that is the first maneuver the examiner should perform. If the patient perceives double vision with one eye occluded, this is monocular diplopia. Monocular diplopia is most often produced by an ocular disorder

that will disrupt the incoming parallel rays of light, preventing them from coming to a point focus on the retina. Instead, a blur circle is formed on the retina and a *ghost image* that is often described as diplopia results. The most frequent causes of monocular diplopia are:

a) Refractive error, especially astigmatism
b) Cataract, usually of the nuclear sclerotic variety
c) Corneal scarring
d) Iris abnormalities, such as atrophy or generous peripheral iridotomies
e) Subluxated lens or implant
f) Non-physiologic causes

The easiest way to document that monocular diplopia is due to a refractive or an anterior segment problem is to use the pinhole. An occluder with multiple pinhole openings from 2-2.5 mm each is placed in front of the patient's symptomatic eye (Figure 9–1). She is then asked if the monocular diplopia is improved or has disappeared. An affirmative answer establishes the anterior segment or a refractive error as the cause of the problem.

2. Determine if misalignment is **comitant** or **incomitant**

If the patient indicates that diplopia is present only with both eyes open, the patient has true **binocular diplopia.** This symptom is almost always due to ocular misalignment. The purpose of this step and the next several steps is to essentially identify isolated or combined cranial nerve (CN) palsies.

A comitant strabismus is one in which

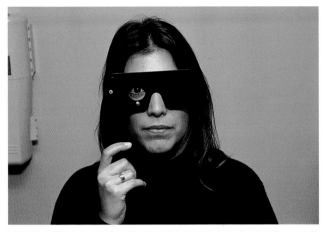

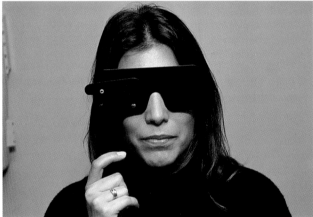

Figure 9–1. *Patient complains of diplopia in the right eye that disappears when the pinhole occluder is placed before the eye.*

the amount of deviation is the same in all directions of gaze and irrespective of which eye is fixating. A strabismus is **incomitant,** when the angle of deviation varies with the direction of gaze or depending on which eye is fixating. Comitant ocular misalignments are usually decompensated congenital deviations. Incomitant misalignments are usually acquired disorders. Certain congenital decompensated phorias e.g., congenital CN IV palsies, may produce incomitant misalignments. The presence of a comitant deviation, particularly when ocular ductions and versions are full (see be-

low) usually indicates a non-neurological cause for the diplopia.

There are several ways to measure the pattern of the ocular misalignment.

Prism Cover Test By introducing prism in front of one eye and utilizing a cover/uncover or alternate cover test, the amount of ocular misalignment is measured in prism diopters (PD). All measurements should be performed in at least six directions of gaze: primary position, right, left, up and down gaze and at near. Oblique gaze and measurements on head tilt are employed under special circumstances. The measurement is then recorded on a chart, which signifies these directions of gaze (Figure 9–2). In the appropriate clinical setting, the ocular misalignment is measured on right and left head tilt. This is usually used when either a CN IV palsy or an ocular tilt reaction is suspected. The patient is seated in the upright position; the head is tilted to the right and then to the left, and the vertical misalignment is measured in the right and left head tilt positions. In CN IV palsies, the vertical misalignment will be greater when the head is tilted toward the side of the palsy.

The **primary deviation** refers to the amount of ocular misalignment measured when the patient is fixating with the non-paretic eye. The **secondary deviation** is the measured angle of deviation when the patient is fixating with the paretic eye. Patients with non-paralytic strabismus do not measure a difference between the primary and secondary deviations; the ocular misalignment is the same when they fix with either eye. The patient with a paralytic strabismus, however, will have a much larger ocular misalignment when the paretic eye is fixing (secondary deviation) and less of a misalignment when the non-paretic eye is fixing (primary deviation) (Figure 9–3). In patients with paralytic strabismus the secondary deviation is always greater than the primary deviation. This is due to Hering's law of equal innervation to yoke muscles.

Red lens or Maddox Rod In this method of measurement, the eyes are dissociated by introducing a red lens or rod in front of one (by convention the right) eye. The patient therefore will see the image (point of light) from each eye as different colors in the case of the red lens test, and as different shapes (a red line and a white point of light) when the Maddox rod is employed (Figure 9–4). If two separate images are perceived, the patient is asked if the red image is to the right or left of the fixation light being viewed at distance. An esotropia will have the red image on the same side as the eye that has the red occluder (uncrossed diplopia). An exotropia, on the other hand, will have the red image on the side opposite to the red occluder (crossed diplopia). In vertical misalignments, the red lens or rod in front of the higher (hypertropic) eye projects the red image as being lower while the red image is seen above the fixation light when the eye behind the red occluder is lower (hypotropia).

The Maddox rod may also be used to measure tortion. This may be done behind the phoropter or by placing the Maddox rod in trial frames. Double Maddox rods (white in front of the left eye, red in front of the right eye) may be employed. The patient (or examiner) turns the adjustment knob on the trial frame or appropriate dial on the phoropter until the two lines are parallel. The amount of tortion is read in degrees directly from the apparatus holding the Maddox rods (Figure 9–5).

3. Examine ductions and versions
    The patient is asked to follow an object horizontally and then vertically. The ocular excursions are judged to be full or limited in one or more directions of gaze. This is then

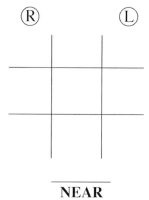

Figure 9–2. *Chart for recording the ocular misalignment in prism diopters in the cardinal positions of gaze.*

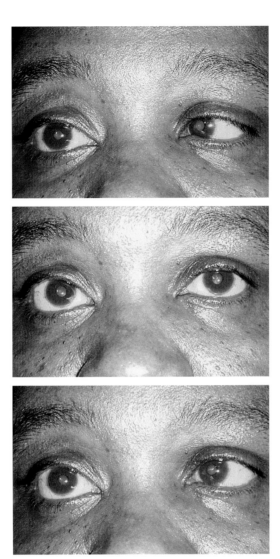

Figure 9–3. Primary and secondary deviation. *Patient has a right CN VI palsy with inability to abduct the right eye (top). The esotropia decreases markedly with the left eye fixing (middle). There is a marked left esotropia with the right eye fixing (bottom).*

recorded either as the percentage of ductional deficit or of the ductional ability (Figure 9–6). At times ductional deficits may not be seen, but "over actions" of muscles may be noted. This is often seen in CN IV palsies where the inferior oblique muscle ipsilateral to the paretic superior oblique muscle tends to overshoot. This is a result of Hering's Law.

4. Examine saccades and pursuits
   On saccadic testing, the patient is asked to look quickly from one direction of gaze into another. For example, right gaze to primary position, or left gaze to primary position. The speed of the saccade is noted, as well as its extent. Normally, patients make refixational movements quickly and in one movement. Saccades may be slowed or ab-

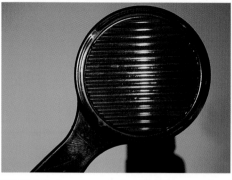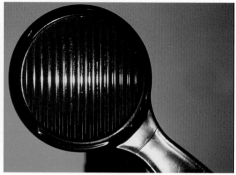

Figure 9–4. *A vertical red line is appreciated when the Maddox rod is placed horizontally and a horizontal line when it is positioned vertically.*

sent, or may occur in a series of smaller movements (hypometric saccades) in order to bring the eye into the required position.

5. Perform forced duction test (if appropriate). Not all ocular misalignments that produce double vision are due to ocular motor paresis. Restrictive ocular myopathies caused by orbital inflammatory disease (myositis) or thyroid related orbitopathy (TRO) are frequent

causes of ocular misalignment and double vision. Likewise, myasthenia gravis (MG) may cause a pattern of double vision that can mimic any isolated muscle palsy, isolated CN palsy, combined CN palsies or supranuclear ocular motility disturbance.

A **forced duction test** (Figure 9–7) should be performed if there is any suspicion that a restrictive myopathy is the cause of the

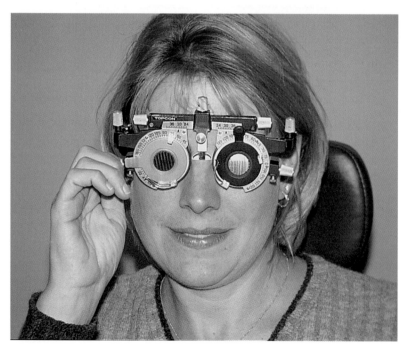

Figure 9–5. *Patient with CN IV palsy rotating red Maddox rod to determine the torsional component.*

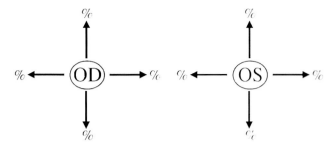

Figure 9–6. *Chart to record ductions in percentages.*

patient's diplopia. The examiner grasps the eye with the restricted duction and attempts to move it into the field of ductional deficit as the patient looks in that direction. The ability to easily move the eye in that direction is a *negative* forced duction test, and indicates that restriction is not present. Perceived difficulty or inability to passively rotate the eye into the direction of ductional deficit is evidence that a restriction exists. This is a *positive* forced duction test and suggests that the cause of the eye movement abnormality is not a neurologic disorder but is most likely due to local orbital disease.

We prefer to perform the forced duction test by anesthetizing the muscle opposite the direction of ductional deficit. For example, with an elevation deficit, we grasp the inferior rectus muscle. This is done with broad forceps after a cotton-tipped applicator soaked with cocaine 10% has been applied over the inferior rectus muscle for two minutes. The patient is asked to look up; the inferior rectus muscle is grasped and the eye is rotated superiorly. The degree of resistance to this passive duction is recorded.

6. Examine lids and pupils.

Other clues to the cause of diplopia may be obtained by observing other aspects of the ocular examination. In all patients who present with diplopia specific attention should be paid to the lid position and the pupillary size. A combination of diplopia and either a lid and/or pupillary abnormality will often provide the examiner with the precise cause of the patient's double vision.

7. Ocular Cephalic Movements

In patients who appear to have bilateral ductional deficits, it is important to determine if this is due to an infranuclear or supranuclear lesion. Supranuclear lesions will produce ductional deficits on voluntary gaze, but by performing dolls head maneuvers, the eyes rotate normally into the field of the ductional deficit. This is often seen in patients with the dorsal midbrain syndrome and progressive supranuclear palsy (PSP). (see p. 198)

8. Nystagmus

Part of the examination of the efferent system is to look for abnormal rhythmic eye movements. If nystagmus is present, the direction of the nystagmus is named by the direction of the fast phase (right-beating, left-beating, etc), and in what cardinal gazes it is present. The amplitude of nystagmus should also be recorded. Tortional nystagmus is recorded as being clockwise or counterclockwise as the examiner looks at the patient, not as the patient's eyes are moving (for example, clockwise nystagmus is when the 12 to 6 o'clock axis rotates towards the examiner's right as the examiner faces the patient).

9. Binocular single vision visual field

When a patient has diplopia, an excellent way to follow progression of the ocular misalignment is by doing binocular single vision visual fields. The patient is seated in front of a bowl kinetic perimeter with both eyes open and is asked to view the central fixation dot. She is then asked to *follow* the III$_4$e light with her eyes only and to indicate when the light

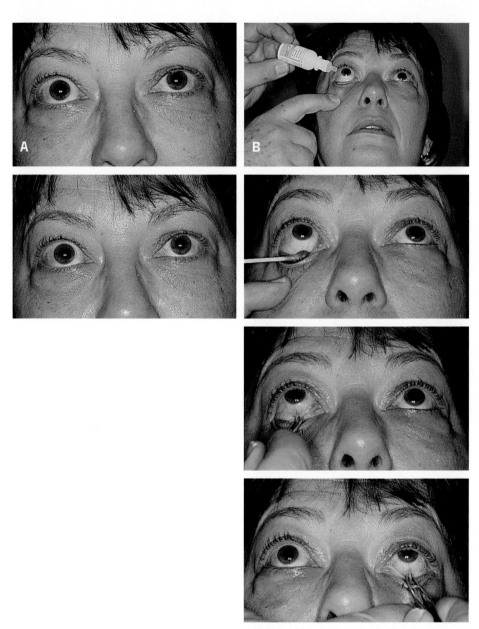

Figure 9–7. Forced Duction Test *A. The patient has right upper lid retraction and injection over the right lateral rectus muscle (top) characteristic of TRO. She cannot elevate either eye (bottom).* ***B.*** *Ophthetic solution is placed into both eyes. A cotton tip applicator soaked in cocaine 10% is placed over the muscle to be grasped for 2 minutes. The body of the muscle opposite to the defective duction is grasped with a broad-based forceps and the patient is asked to look in the direction of defective gaze while the examiner attempts to rotate the eye in that direction. Resistance to passive rotation of the eye is a positive test. The fellow eye is tested in a similar manner.*

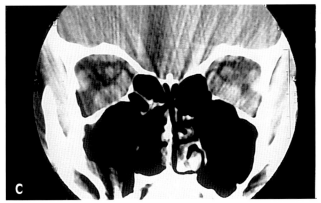

Figure 9-7. *(Continued)* **Forced Duction Test** *C. Coronal CT scan showing enlarged inferior rectus muscles bilaterally consistent with TRO.*

switches from being single to double. The points are plotted so that a diagram of the area in which the patient sees single is created. This diagram may then be used on subsequent visits to determine if the patient's field of single vision is changing (Figure 9–8).

Ocular Motility Disturbances without diplopia: Some patients present with oc-ular motility disturbances, but do not have diplopia. This may be because of poor vision in one or both eyes, or because the ocular motility disturbance has not produced an ocular misalignment. In these patients, the examination consists of evaluation of ductions and version, saccades and pursuits, forced ductions and evaluation for MG.

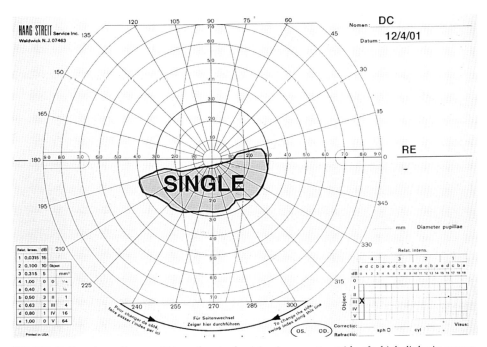

Figure 9-8. *A small area of binocular single vision is present outside of which diplopia occurs.*

Chapter 10

OCULAR MISALIGNMENT AND OTHER OCULAR MOTOR DISORDERS

CRANIAL NERVE III PALSY

Cranial nerve III (CN III) innervates the superior, inferior, medial recti, and the inferior oblique muscles. It also innervates the levator palpebrae superioris and carries with it the parasympathetic innervation to the pupil. Involvement of CN III will produce a symptom complex that involves one or several of these muscles and usually results in double vision.

Anatomy

Cranial nerve III originates in the midbrain from subnuclei. The subnuclei give rise to the fascicles of each of the extraocular muscles. The superior rectus subnuclei are crossed so that the left superior rectus subnucleus eventually innervates the right superior rectus muscle. Another peculiarity of the nuclear structure of CN III is that the nucleus for the upper lids is a single midline structure innervating the levator muscles of both lids. As CN III leaves the brainstem and enters the cavernous sinus, it divides anatomically into a superior and inferior division. The superior division contains the superior rectus and levator innervation, while the inferior division contains the rest of the innervation for CN III. There is convincing evidence that the functional organization into a superior and inferior division occurs before the anatomic division occurs in the cavernous sinus.

Etiology and Pathophysiology

Cranial III neuropathy may be caused by a variety of processes, but the most frequent causes

are either microvascular infarction of the nerve itself or compression. Microvascular infarction occurs in older patients (over 45 years of age) and is due to occlusion of the vaso nevorum. This infarction involves the axial portion of CN III. Since the pupillary fibers are on the periphery of the nerve, the pupil is not involved by the axial infarction in microvascular disease. These patients often have identifiable risk factors such as diabetes mellitus, hypertension, atherosclerosis, and hyperlipidemia.

Compressive CN III palsies may be produced by tumors or aneurysms. The clinical syndrome of an aneurismal CN III palsy is an important one because it is a medical emergency. The patient will usually present with a painful isolated CN III palsy. This is usually due to a posterior communicating (PCOM) artery aneurysm. The aneurysm exerts pressure from the outside, thus the pupillary fibers are often involved early and the CN III palsy is characterized by ptosis, ocular misalignment, and, usually, a dilated pupil.

Clinical Characteristics

See Figure 10–1.

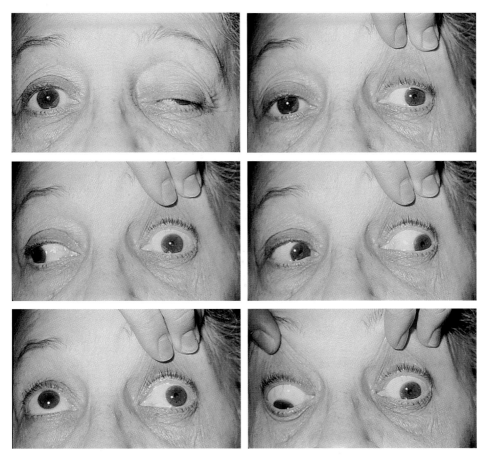

Figure 10–1. *Left upper lid ptosis is almost complete and there is an exotropia when the left lid is elevated (top row). The left eye cannot be adducted, elevated, or depressed. The pupils are equal in size.*

Symptoms

1. Pain may be present with CN III palsies due to microvascular infarction or compression. It *does not* distinguish between the two causes.
2. Ptosis may be complete or incomplete.
3. Diplopia is usually oblique in nature.

Signs

1. Ptosis may be complete or incomplete.
2. Ophthalmoplegia: there is usually an ex-otropia in primary position with defective adduction, elevation, and depression of the eye.
3. Anisocoria (Figure 10–2) occurs with compression, otherwise the pupils are normal.

The presence of anisocoria and a dilated pupil is critical to the diagnosis of an aneurismal CN III palsy. Thus, any patient diagnosed with a lesion of CN III must have the pupil evaluated. The *rule of the pupil* states that in a *complete* CN III palsy, the pupil will be normal if the cause is microvascular infarction, but will be dilated and less reactive to light if the lesion is compressive, especially by a PCOM

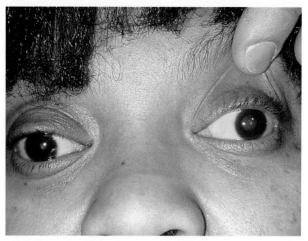

Figure 10–2. *Patient has a left CN III palsy with a dilated pupil.*

aneurysm. There are certain caveats to invoking the rule of the pupil.

- It may be invoked only in the presence of a complete CN III palsy. It would be unwise to invoke this rule in incomplete or partial palsies (Figure 10–3).
- It has been reported that the pupil may initially be uninvolved with PCOM aneurysms, with the anisocoria developing at any time within 5 days of the start of diplopia.

Investigations

Once the CN III palsy has been diagnosed, the next step is to determine if the palsy is isolated. An associated CN VI deficit is usually easily seen but an accompanying CN IV palsy may be less obvious. The primary action of CN IV is depression in adduction, however in the presence of a complete CN III palsy, the eye cannot be adducted to test for CN IV integrity. The determination is made by looking for the secondary action of CN IV, intorsion of the globe. The patient is instructed to look down while the examiner looks for intorsion. Its absence indicates CN IV paresis (Figure 10–4).

The investigation of an isolated CN III palsy will depend on the age of the patient, the completeness of the palsy, and the state of the pupil. Guidelines for investigations using these factors are in Table 10–1.

1. Aneurysms are extraordinarily rare in children under 10 years of age but ophthalmoplegic migraine is a frequent cause of CN III palsies with pupillary involvement; thus, the rationale for subjecting children with CN III palsies to MRI and MRA, but not catheter angiography.
2. Patients in the vasculopathic age range with risk factors and no pupillary involvement require no investigation except to identify those risk factors if none are known to be present, for example, determination of glucose status and blood pressure. However, if the pupil is involved, the patient should have an MRI and MRA, and if negative, because the chances of a PCOM aneurysm are still high, catheter angiography.
3. Patients younger than the vasculopathic age range but older than 10 years require MRI and MRA to rule out tumors or aneurysms even if the pupil is normal. If the pupil is abnormal, however, catheter angiography should be performed even if the MRI and MRA are negative. If all imaging tests are unrevealing, then further hematologic and spinal fluid investigations are recommended.

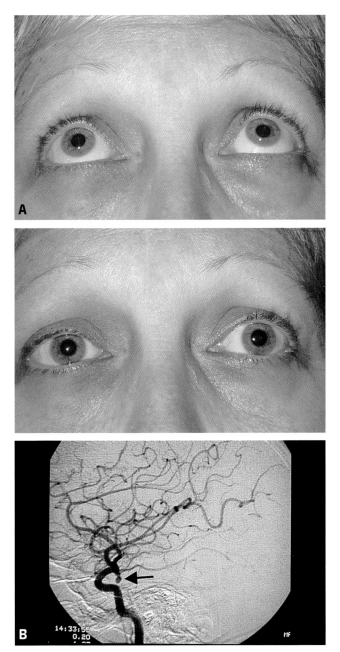

Figure 10-3. *A. There is a small left exotropia and hypertropia in primary gaze with the right eye fixing and slight ptosis of the right upper lid. Upgaze is minimally less OD. The pupils are equal.* ***B.*** *MRI, MRA, and lumbar puncture were normal, but because of the patient's young age and the presence of headaches, catheter arteriography was done and revealed a right PCOM aneurysm* (arrow).

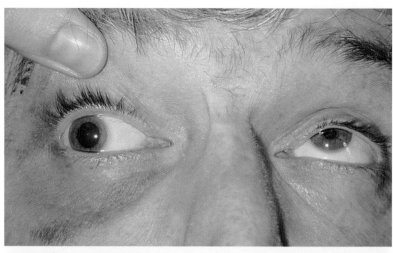

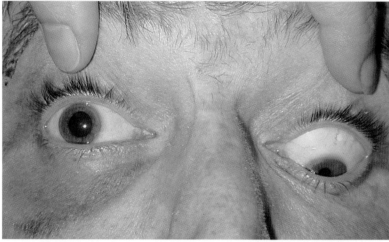

Figure 10–4. *Patient has a right pupil involving CN III following trauma. Note that the conjunctival blood vessel below the right upper lid is in the same position on both up- and downgaze. This lack of intorsion on attempted downgaze indicates a paresis of CN IV.*

TABLE 10–1. INVESTIGATION OF THIRD CRANIAL NERVE PALSIES

	Under 10 Years	11–50 Years	Over 50 Years
Anisocoria less than 2 mm	MRI MRA	MRI, MRA If negative, perform medical work-up	Observe without imaging*
Anisocoria greater than 2 mm	MRI MRA**	MRI, MRA If negative, catheter angiography	MRI, MRA If negative, catheter angiography

* Determine the status of the blood pressure, glucose metabolism, and the presence of other medical risk factors.
** Catheter angiography may be justified if these tests are negative.

Differential Diagnosis

A variety of entities produce ocular motor syndromes that can be confused with complete or partial CN III palsies.

1. Thyroid related orbitopathy often produces abnormalities of the medial and inferior rectus muscles. Lid retraction, if present, and a positive forced duction test will establish the correct diagnosis (see Fig 9-7).
2. Myasthenia gravis also may simulate any pattern of a CN III palsy including ptosis. The pupil is never involved in MG and the lid and ocular motility disturbances are variable.
3. Orbital trauma can produce an upgaze defect as the result of entrapment of the inferior rectus muscle or as part of a traumatic orbital apex/superior orbital fissure syndrome (see p. XX). Vertical diplopia also can occur following cataract surgery (Figure 10–5). The cause of the superior rectus "weakness" is actually trauma to the inferior rectus muscle and/or its nerve by the retrobulbar injection. These misalignments may resolve over several months but at times require corrective surgery.

4. Orbital inflammation involving the extraocular muscles may resemble a partial CN III palsy. Orbital imaging will reveal the true cause of the ocular misalignment (Figure 10–6).

Clinical Course

1. Vasculopathic CN III palsies will resolve spontaneously over a period of 6 to 12 weeks. It is very uncommon for there to be residual diplopia.
2. Cranial nerve palsies due to compression will resolve if the compression is removed, or will resolve in a pattern called *aberrant regeneration*.
3. The conditions that should prompt investigation of a CN III palsy under observation are listed in Table 10–2.

Aberrant Regeneration of Cranial Nerve III

Aberrant regeneration of CN III (Figure 10–7), a stereotypic pattern, most often follows an acute CN III palsy due to a PCOM aneurysm or

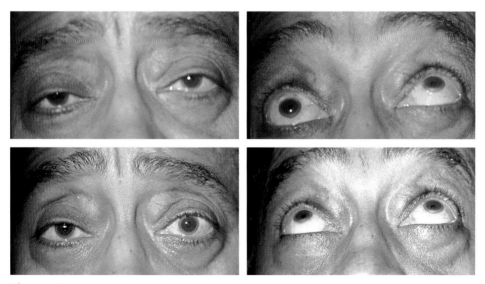

Figure 10–5. *Vertical diplopia appeared after cataract surgery OD with retrobulbar anesthesia. Right upper lid ptosis and poor upgaze (top row) improved over several months (bottom row).*

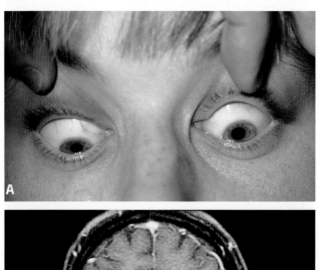

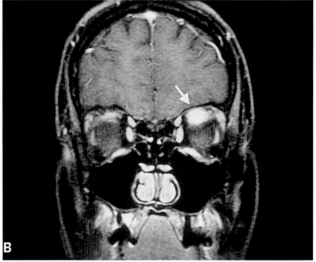

Figure 10-6. *A. Diplopia present on downgaze due to inability to depress the left eye.*
B. Coronal MRI scan reveals enlargement and increased enhancement of the left superior rectus,
levator complex (arrow). The forced duction test was positive.

pituitary apoplexy. The ptosis resolves completely or is minimally evident. The eye usually will not elevate or depress well, but adduction usually is restored. The pupil is nonreactive to light, but will react when the patient adducts the eye. The lid shows a synkinetic movement on adduction and downgaze where the interpalpebral fissure widens. This widening of the interpalpebral fissure on down gaze is known as the pseudo-Graefe sign.

Aberrant regeneration is a pattern of resolution in compressive or traumatic CN III palsies.

It should never be attributed to a vasculopathic CN III palsy.

Primary Aberrant Regeneration Some patients never experience an acute CN III palsy, but develop a slowly progressive form of CN III aberrant regeneration. Slow growing compressive lesions, usually within the cavernous sinus, produce this syndrome. These lesions are usually meningiomas or cavernous sinus aneurysms, although other causes have been reported.

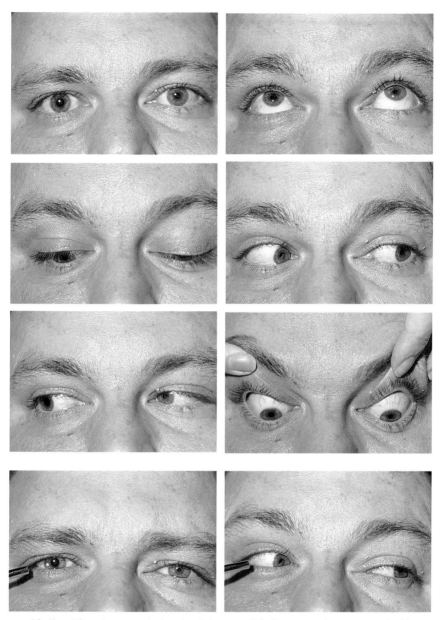

Figure 10–7. *There is no ptosis, but the right upper lid elevates on downgaze and adduction. There is a slight deficit on elevation of OD. The right pupil is larger and does not constrict to light, but does so on adduction and depression of OD. The patient had pituitary apoplexy 6 months before with a complete CN III palsy OD.*

TABLE 10–2. WHEN TO INVESTIGATE A CRANIAL NERVE III PALSY UNDER OBSERVATION

The pupil dilates

An incomplete CN III palsy progresses after 1 week

Other neurologic signs or symptoms develop

Aberrant regeneration appears

There is no resolution in 3 months

Brainstem Lesions

Lesions in the brainstem can produce several specific syndromes of CN III (see Table 10–3). When the CN III nucleus is affected, a variety of ocular motility patterns are observed.

1. Unilateral CN III palsy with bilateral ptosis and contralateral superior rectus paresis.
2. Bilateral CN III palsies without ptosis.
3. Bilateral ptosis alone.
4. Any isolated palsy of a muscle innervated by CN III

   Nuclear CN III palsies are extraordinarily infrequent.

TABLE 10–3. MIDBRAIN FASCICULAR THIRD CRANIAL NERVE PALSIES

Syndrome	Signs	Location of Lesion
Weber's	CN III palsy	Corticospinal tracts
	Contralateral hemiplegia	Cerebral peduncle
Benedikt	CN III palsy	Red nucleus
	Contralateral ataxia and involuntary movements	
Nothnagel	CN III palsy	Brachium conjunctivum
	Ipsilateral ataxia	

CRANIAL NERVE IV PALSY

Cranial nerve IV (CN IV) innervates only the superior oblique muscle, which depresses the eye in adduction and intorts the eye. Cranial nerve IV is the only cranial nerve that exits the brainstem dorsally. It also decussates so that the right nucleus of CN IV will eventually innervate the left superior oblique muscle. Cranial nerve IV is enveloped in the anterior medullary vellum where it is vulnerable to head trauma.

Etiology

1. Head trauma
2. Microvascular infarction
3. Congenital
4. Other causes such as tumors, multiple sclerosis, and inflammation are less frequent

Clinical Characteristics

Symptoms

1. Diplopia is oblique in nature.
2. Difficulty reading or walking down stairs.

Signs

1. Vertical misalignment: the ocular misalignment is usually a hypertropia ipsilateral to the side of the cranial nerve involvement. It is worse on gaze to the contralateral side and on ipsilateral head tilt. (For example, a right CN IV palsy produces a right hypertropia worse in left gaze and right head tilt).

   The method to most easily detect this misalignment is the Parks Three Step Test, which determines by using cover-uncover test if (Figure 10–8):
   • there is a hypertropia in primary position,
   • the hypertropia increases in left or right gaze, and
   • the hypertropia increases on head tilt to either side (Bielschowsky head-tilt test).
2. The head is tilted away from the side of the cranial nerve palsy. The chin may be depressed (Figure 10–9 top).
3. Overaction of the ipsilateral inferior oblique muscle, the antagonist of the paretic superior oblique muscle, is demonstrable (Figure 10–9 middle).
4. Excyclotorsion may be documented using:
   • The double Maddox rod or Lancaster red-green glasses (Figure 10–9 C).
   • Ophthalmoscopy: normally, the fovea is 0.3-mm below imaginary line drawn through the geometric center of the optic disc. With direct ophthalmoscopy, the fovea will appear *lower* if excyclotorsion is present (Figure 10–10).
5. Vertical fusional amplitude: the normal vertical fusional range is 1 to 3 prism diopters. Patients with a congenital CN IV palsy have an increased range of fusional amplitudes.

Investigations

In the presence of an isolated CN IV palsy, a history of head trauma should be sought. If no trauma occurred, an isolated CN IV palsy in a patient over 45 years is assumed to be vasculopathic in nature. Patients younger than the vasculopathic age group should undergo neuroimaging. Congenital CN IV palsies may become manifest later in life. These patients complain of intermittent diplopia that becomes more frequent and more prolonged. Examination reveals increased vertical fusional amplitudes, which establishes the diagnosis of a congenital process. Examining old family photographs likewise may reveal a long-standing head tilt, another clue to the congenital nature of the strabismus. In patients with increased vertical fusional amplitudes, no further investigations are required. Vertical fusional ampli-

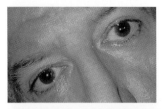
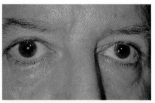
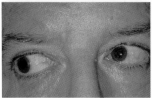
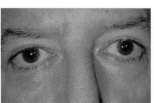
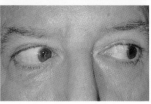

Figure 10–8. *There is an intermittent left hypertropia of 10 PD in primary gaze. It increases dramatically in right gaze due to an overaction of the left inferior oblique muscle. It is larger on left than on right head tilt* (top row).

tudes should be measured in all patients with a CN IV palsy.

Course

1. Patients in the vasculopathic age group with an isolated CN IV palsy and normal vertical fusional amplitudes require investigation for risk factors (eg. diabetes mellitus and hypertension). These patients then may be observed since most of these palsies will resolve spontaneously within 6 to 12 weeks.
2. Patients with traumatic CN IV palsies also may be observed. The misalignment, however, may take longer to resolve.

Treatment

Prisms may be tried, but because of the incomitant and, at times the torsional nature of this ocular misalignment, they are often not successful. Surgical realignment of the eyes is often the final solution for these patients.

Bilateral Cranial Nerve IV Palsies

Trauma often produces bilateral CN IV palsies. The bilaterality of the process may be masked and patients will sometimes appear to have a unilateral palsy. Clues to bilateral involvement include:

1. Large cyclorotational misalignment: patients with an apparent "unilateral" CN IV palsy but with excyclotorsion >15 degrees should be suspected of having bilateral CN IV palsies.
2. V-pattern esotropia.
3. Alternating hypertropia (right hypertropia on left gaze and left hypertropia on right gaze).

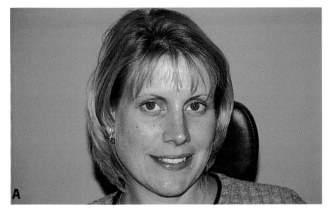

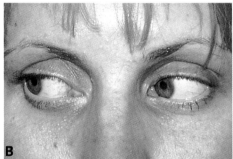

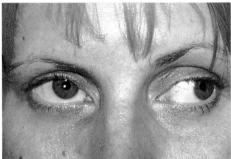

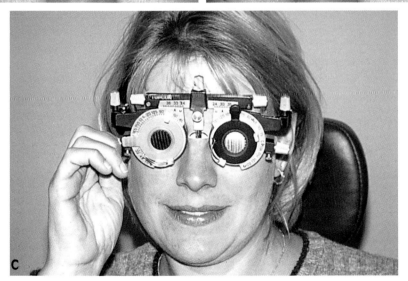

Figure 10–9. *A. Patient with right CN IV palsy with a left head tilt and a chin down position. B. Right gaze is normal but there is marked overaction of the right inferior oblique muscle in left gaze. C. Excyclotorsion is measured with the double Maddox rod.*

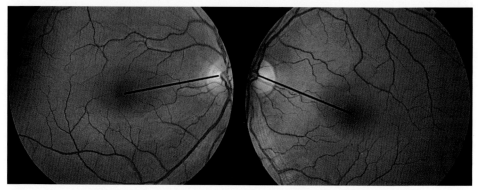

Figure 10–10. *Fundus photograph shows the normal position of the macula in relation to the optic disc in the right eye (left) and the lower position of the macula in the exotorted left eye (right) of a patient with a left CN IV palsy.*

CRANIAL NERVE VI PALSY

Cranial nerve (CN) VI has one of the longest intracranial courses. Involvement of this nerve throughout its extranuclear course results in an esotropia and an ipsilateral abduction deficit.

Anatomy

The anatomical peculiarity of CN VI is that a lesion in its nucleus will *not* produce an isolated ipsilateral CN VI palsy. The abducens nucleus contains, in addition to cells that give origin to CN VI, interneurons, which give origin to fibers that eventually end in the contralateral medial rectus subnucleus of CN III. This anatomic arrangement ensures conjugate horizontal eye movements, however, it also means that a lesion involving the CN VI nucleus will produce not an ipsilateral abduction deficit, but an ipsilateral gaze palsy.

Cranial nerve VI also lies in proximity to certain other structures throughout its fascicular and peripheral course. It is in close proximity to CN VII in the brainstem and is contained along with CN III, IV, and V within the cavernous sinus. Lesions in these areas are likely to produce combined cranial nerve palsies instead of an isolated CN VI palsy.

Etiology

The more frequent causes of CN VI palsies are:

1. Vasculopathic (microvascular infarction)
2. Trauma
3. Meningitic processes (inflammatory, infectious, and neoplastic)
4. Mass lesions
5. Increased intracranial pressure from any cause
6. Multiple sclerosis
7. Post lumbar puncture or spinal anesthesia
8. Stroke
9. Congenital

Clinical Characteristics

Symptoms

1. Double vision
2. Pain around the eye at times, depending on the cause

Signs

1. Esotropia is usually present in primary gaze and increases in lateral gaze (Figure 10–11). The esotropia is worse when the paretic eye is fixating (primary and secondary deviation; see p. 111, Figure 9–3). This differs from a congenital esotropia, in which the measurement of the esotropia is the same with either eye fixating.
2. Abduction defect may be partial or total.
3. The saccades in the direction of the paresis is usually slowed.

Congenital Cranial Nerve VI Palsy

Isolated congenital CN VI palsies usually result from birth trauma.

Several syndromes occur that combine congenital CN VI palsies with other features.

Möbius Syndrome Children with Möbius syndrome have mask-like facies due to facial diplegia and mostly bilateral, but at times unilateral, abduction deficits. They may have no esotropia in primary position. Complete absence of horizontal gaze may be a feature of the disorder.

Duane's Retraction Syndrome Of the three types of Duane's retraction syndrome, type I consists of an isolated abduction deficit, which may be unilateral or bilateral. These patients do

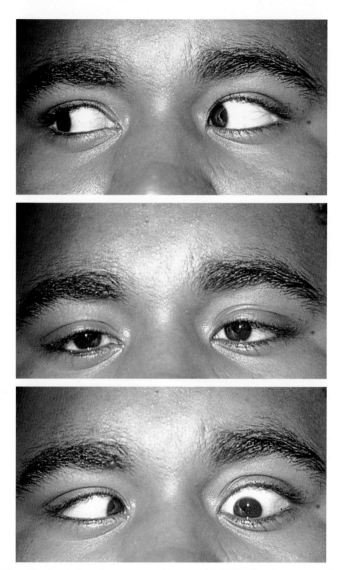

Figure 10–11. *Esotropia in primary gaze with a total left CN VI palsy appeared after lumbar puncture. The ocular motility returned to normal within 4 months.*

not usually have an esotropia in primary position and do not appreciate diplopia. They may, however, have abnormal eyelid movements with the lid retracting on ipsilateral adduction (Figure 10–12).

Duane's retraction syndrome has actually been shown to be due to a prenatal lesion in the CN VI nucleus. The nuclear cells that give rise to the ipsilateral abducens nerve are absent. A portion of cranial nerve III, therefore, innervates the lateral rectus muscle thus producing the cocontracture that results in retraction of the globe that characterizes Duane's syndrome.

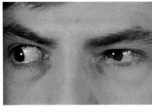 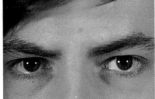 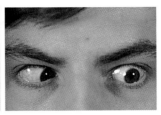

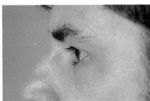 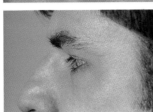

Figure 10–12. *There is an esotropia in primary gaze with a left abduction deficit. On right gaze, the left lid fissure narrows and the left eye retracts (side view).*

Investigations

The type and extent of the investigation will depend on multiple factors including the patient's age, associated ophthalmologic and neurologic findings, and the uni- or bilaterality of the CN VI palsies.

1. Patients over 45 years of age who develop a CN VI palsy will often have a so-called *vasculopathic* cause for their deficit. This is a vascular occlusion to the CN VI itself. These infarcts in the nerve are usually sudden in onset and painless, although pain at times may be a feature of an isolated vasculopathic CN VI palsy. These palsies are usually self-limiting and tend to resolve within 3 months. In a patient over 45 years of age who has an *isolated* CN VI palsy, and who has vasculopathic risk factors such as diabetes mellitus, hypertension, hypercholesterolemia and so forth, a workup may be deferred. If the CN VI palsy resolves in the specified period of time, a vasculopathic etiology may be inferred. It is recommended that investigations, including MRI, be performed if:
   - The CN VI palsy does not resolve within the 3-month period of time (Figure 10–13).
   - The esotropia progresses after 2 weeks from its onset.
   - Other signs or symptoms develop. *metastic*
   - We also routinely image anyone with a previous history of malignancy even if the CN VI is isolated (Figure 10–14).
2. Although vasculopathic CN VI palsies can be recurrent either on the same or opposite side, the bilateral simultaneous occurrence of CN VI palsies should never be considered vasculopathic in origin. In this circumstance, a workup for other causes should be undertaken.
3. In all patients with unilateral or bilateral CN VI palsy, ophthalmoscopy with examination of the optic discs looking for papilledema is required. Increased intracranial pressure from any cause can produce unilateral or bilateral CN VI palsies as a nonlocalizing sign of the increased intracranial pressure.
4. Patients under age 45 years who present with acquired uni- or bilateral CN VI palsies require investigation. If there is no preceding history of trauma or any other obvious cause for the CN VI palsy, a complete medical history and general neurologic examination should be conducted. MRI is a critical part of the workup in these patients and should be performed on all of them. If the MRI is unrevealing, a lumbar puncture with examination of the cerebrospinal fluid should be considered.

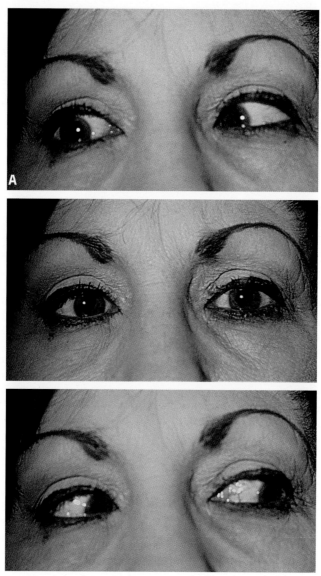

Figure 10–13. *A. Esotropia and right abduction deficit began 6 months before, but has not resolved.*

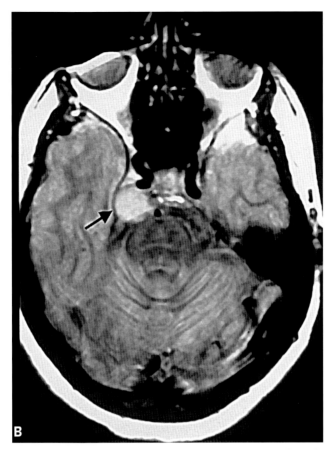

Figure 10–13. *(continued)* **B.** *Axial MRI reveals enhancing mass in the right cavernous sinus* (arrow).

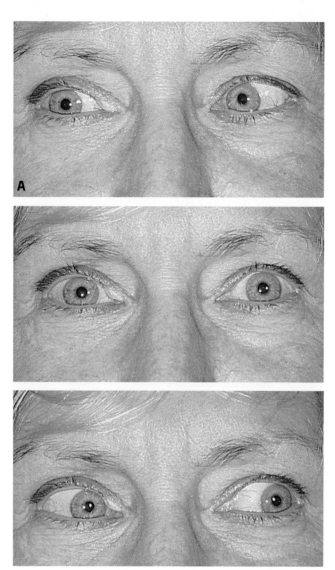

Figure 10–14. *A.* *A 58-year-old woman with an esotropia of 4 PD in her primary gaze and 14 PD on right gaze with a right abduction deficit. Her examination was otherwise unremarkable, but because she had breast cancer 10 years before, an MRI was performed.*

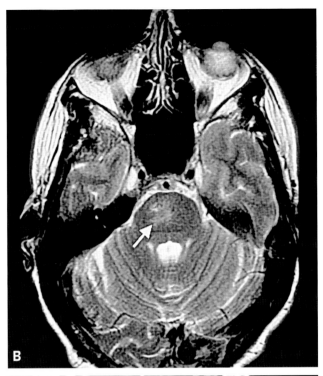

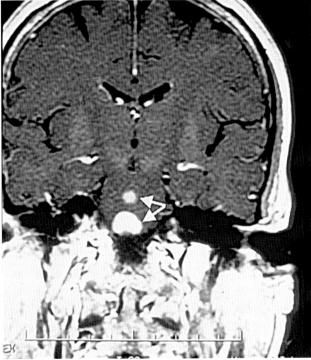

Figure 10–14. (*continued*) *B. Axial and coronal MRI shows two areas of enhancement in the pons* (arrows). *There also were asymptomatic multiple metastatic enhancing lesions in the cerebellum and frontal and temporal lobes.*

Treatment

Treatment of the CN VI palsy obviously depends on its cause. In the isolated vasculopathic scenario, controlling the risk factors might prevent a recurrence of the problem, but will not result in a more prompt resolution of the esotropia.

Treatment of the esotropia itself is similar to that for other forms of ocular misalignment, that is, patching, prisms, or surgery if the ocular misalignment persists.

Special Forms of CN VI palsy

Foville's syndrome is due to involvement of the pontine tegmentum (dorsolateral pons) and consists of:

Ipsilateral

1. CN VI palsy or gaze palsy
2. CN VII palsy
3. Horner's syndrome
4. Analgesia of the face
5. Peripheral deafness
6. Loss of taste to anterior two thirds of the tongue

Millard-Gubler Syndrome is due to involvement of the ventral paramedian pons and consists of

Ipsilateral

1. CN VI palsy
2. CN VII palsy

Contralateral hemiplegia

Pseudo Cranial Nerve VI Palsies

All abduction defects are not CN VI palsies. A variety of other disorders can produce abduction defects, including:

1. Duane's retraction syndrome (see above)
2. Thyroid related orbitopathy (Figure 10–15)
3. Orbital inflammatory disease (myositis, pseudotumor) (Figure 10–16)
4. Myasthenia gravis
5. Medial rectus muscle entrapment
6. Spasm of the near reflex (SNR). Patients with SNR usually have an intermittent esotropia. This is produced by the patient voluntarily activating the near triad of convergence, accommodation, and pupillary miosis. Every time the esotropia and abduction defect occur, the pupils will become miotic (Figure 10–17). Spasm of the near reflex is rarely due to organic disease.

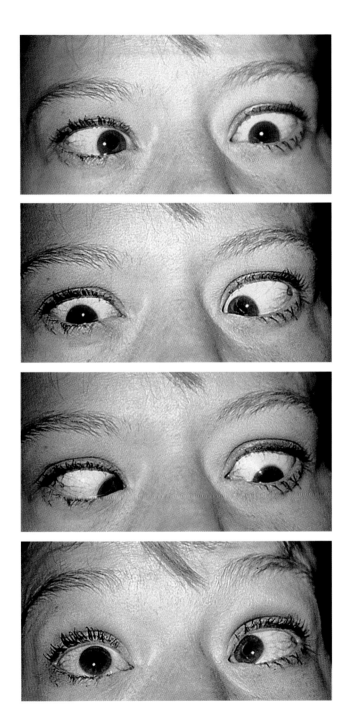

Figure 10–15. *There is a large esotropia in primary gaze (top) with inability to abduct either eye. The clues to the diagnosis of TRO are the lid retraction, the characteristic injection over the lateral rectus muscles and inability to look up with either eye (bottom).*

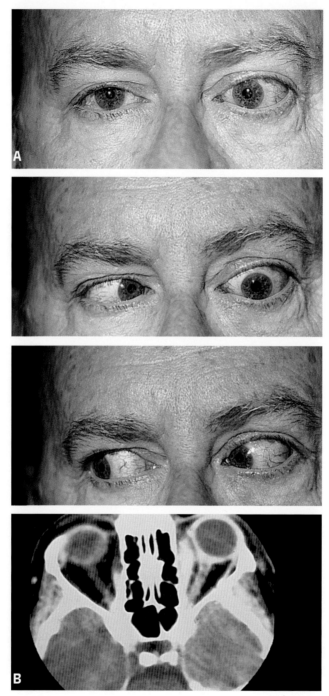

Figure 10-16. *A. Esotropia in primary gaze with absent abduction left eye. The left eye is injected.* ***B.*** *Axial CT scan shows an enlarged, enhancing left medial rectus muscle.*

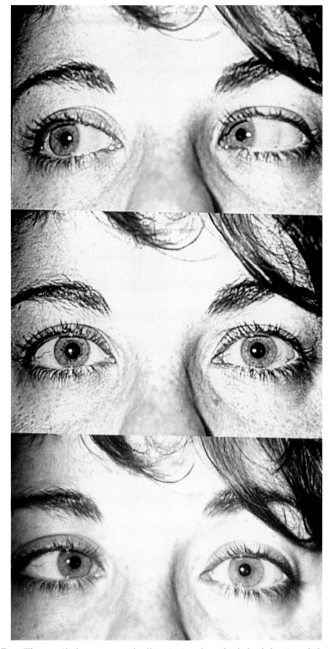

Figure 10–17. *The pupils become markedly miotic when the left abduction defect appears* (bottom).

MULTIPLE CRANIAL NERVE PALSIES

The guidelines for the investigation of CN III, IV, or VI palsies are based largely on their being isolated. The simultaneous presence of more than one CN palsy, or other neurologic signs or symptoms, implies the involvement of different anatomic regions and by and large, the presence of different disease processes than those that produce isolated CN palsies. Associated neurologic findings that accompany the CN palsy help point to the localization of the disease process. For example, a CN III palsy combined with a contralateral hemiparesis indicates a brainstem lesion.

The simultaneous presence of two or more cranial neuropathies requires the clinician to determine if one or multiple lesions are causing the clinical signs. Most of the lesions that produce multiple CN palsies involve the peripheral nerves, whereas lesions producing other neurologic problems, e.g., hemiparesis or contralateral tremor associated with cranial nerve palsies will be found in the brainstem. Cranial nerves III, IV, and VI come together in close proximity in the cavernous sinus, and in this local a single lesion may affect more than one of them.

Cavernous Sinus Syndrome

The cavernous sinus is a venous structure on either side of the pituitary gland. The lateral wall of the sinus contains CN III, IV, and V. Cranial nerve VI traverses the body of the cavernous sinus relatively isolated from the other cranial nerves. The internal carotid artery occupies the central portion of the cavernous sinus (Figure 10–18). The ocular sympathetic fibers destined for the iris dilator muscle are also contained in this portion of the cavernous sinus. A lesion in the cavernous sinus may produce involvement of any of the cranial nerves or other structures contained therein.

Mass lesions in the cavernous sinus (tumors or aneurysms) may at times produce an isolated CN VI palsy. Because of its location within the body

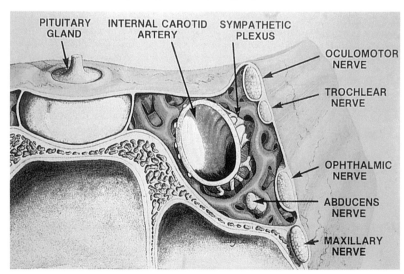

Figure 10–18. *Schematic of cavernous sinus anatomy. (Reprinted from Survey of Ophthalmology vol 27, Kline LB, The Tolosa Hunt Syndrome, pg 79–95, 1982 with permission from Elsevier Science).*

of the cavernous sinus and not within its dural walls, an isolated CN VI palsy may be the first, and at times, the only sign of cavernous sinus disease (see p. XX). More frequently, however, patients with cavernous sinus lesions present with an ocular motility disturbance that is a combination of involvement of CN III, IV, and VI, and often with symptoms attributable to CN V.

Etiology

Any lesion in the cavernous sinus may produce the so-called *cavernous sinus syndrome*. The most frequent causes are:

1. Meningiomas
2. Intracavernous aneurysms
3. Extension of parachiasmal or skull-based mass lesions into the cavernous sinus, for example, pituitary apoplexy
4. Metastatic lesions (Figure 10–19)
5. Inflammation or infection: for example, sarcoidosis, syphilis, mucormycosis (Figure 10–20), herpes zoster, or idiopathic granulomatous inflammation (Tolosa-Hunt syndrome)
6. Arteriovenous fistula (carotid-cavernous or dural) (Figure 10–21)
7. Cavernous sinus thrombosis (Figure 10–22)

Clinical Characteristics

Symptoms

1. Diplopia may be caused by a combination of CN III, IV, and VI, or at times an isolated CN VI palsy.
2. Pain (often severe) or numbness in the distribution of CN V.
3. Lid malposition may be secondary to lid edema from venous engorgement produced by a cavernous sinus mass, or may be due to a ptosis produced by concomitant Horner's syndrome or CN III involvement.
4. Anisocoria may be due to a CN III palsy, Horner's syndrome, or both. If both are present, the pupil may be small or mid-dilated and poorly reactive. This appearance is virtually pathognomonic of a cavernous sinus lesion.

Signs

1. An ocular motility pattern with or without lid and pupillary signs indicating combined involvement of CN III, IV, and VI.
2. Decreased sensation over the distribution of CN V_1 and V_2.
3. Ocular sympathetic paresis (Horner's Syndrome). The combination of an isolated CN VI paresis and Horner's syndrome may suggest an intracavernous aneurysm or another lesion in the body of the sinus. This is because the sympathetic fibers leave the internal carotid artery within the cavernous sinus and join briefly with CN VI before separating and fusing with the ophthalmic division of CN V.

Investigations

The simultaneous presence of two or more CN palsies requires that a MRI scan be performed. If the clinical syndrome involves a combination of CN III, IV, and VI, the cavernous sinus must be imaged.

SUPERIOR ORBITAL FISSURE SYNDROME

The anterior most border of the cavernous sinus is the superior orbital fissure. The clinical signs and symptoms of involvement of this area are identical to the cavernous sinus syndrome with one exception. With lesions of the posterior cavernous sinus, CN V_3 may be involved, whereas this branch is not present in the superior orbital fissure.

ORBITAL APEX SYNDROME

Immediately in front of the superior orbital fissure is the orbital apex. Cranial nerves III, IV, V, and VI may be involved here as well. However, since the optic nerve is contained in the orbit, an orbital apex syndrome must be suspected when signs of an optic neuropathy accompany cranial nerve ocular motility disturbances. Proptosis is another sign of an orbital apex syndrome.

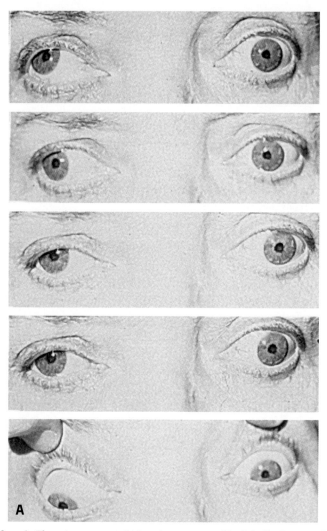

Figure 10–19. *A. There is an exotropia in primary gaze with globally decreased ductions.*

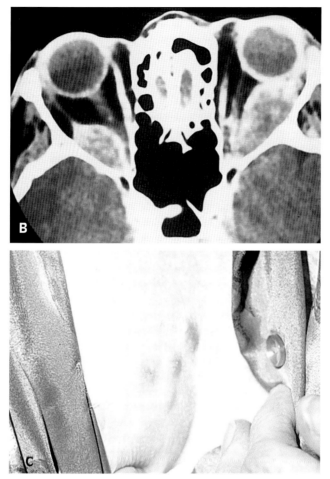

Figure 10–19. (*continued*) **B.** *CT scan reveals masses in each orbit involving the lateral rectus muscles.* **C.** *The patient had breast cancer with metastasis to the chest wall as well as the orbits.*

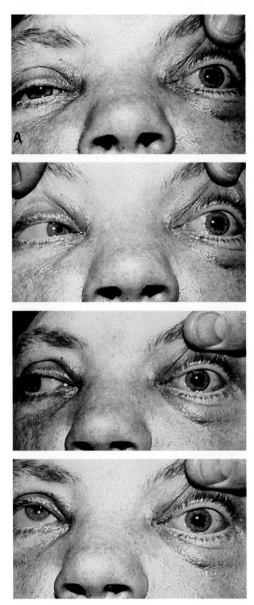

Figure 10–20. *A. Left ptosis and total ophthalmoplegia (downgaze not shown). The patient also had a retinal artery occlusion.*

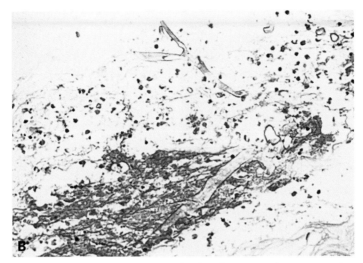

Figure 10–20. *(continued)* **B.** *Non-septate hyphae diagnostic of mucormycosis were identified on orbital biopsy.*

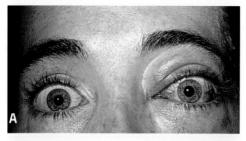

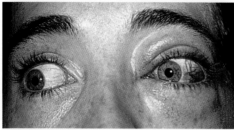

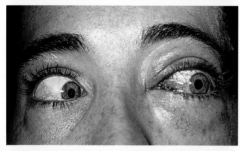

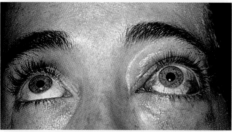

Figure 10–21. *A. The eyes are straight in primary gaze, but there is decreased adduction, abduction, depression (not shown), and elevation of the left eye. There are typical arteriolized conjunctival blood vessels of a carotid cavernous fistula (CCF). B. Axial CT scan shows a greatly enlarged left superior ophthalmic vein (SOV). C. Color Doppler reveals reversal of flow in the left SOV (it appears red instead of its normal blue color).*

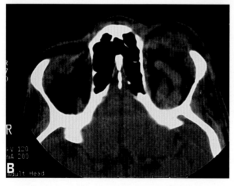

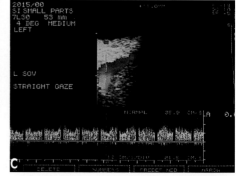

Lesions of the orbit may produce ocular motor disturbances that resemble multiple CN palsies. Thyroid-related orbitopathy is the most frequent cause (see p. XX) but any orbital lesion can produce a similar clinical picture.

OTHER CAUSES OF MULTIPLE CRANIAL NERVE PALSIES

The clinical abnormalities found in the cavernous sinus, superior orbital fissure, and orbital apex syndromes are all ipsilateral. However, simultaneous involvement of more than one cranial nerve on opposite sides may occur. In this situation, one should suspect a more diffuse disease process that involves the meninges or the cerebrospinal fluid. MRI scanning looking for dural enhancement followed by lumbar puncture should be the first investigations performed.

Although it is possible to have the simultaneous involvement of more than one cranial nerve on a vasculopathic basis, this is extraordinarily rare and must remain a diagnosis of exclusion.

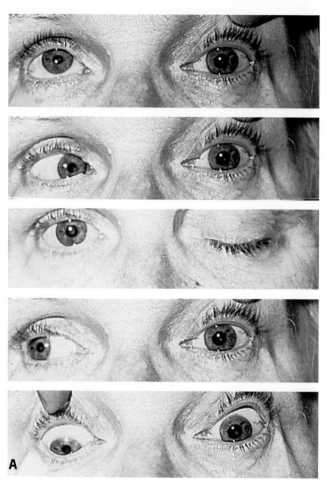

Figure 10–22. *A. Total left ophthalmoplegia. The pupil is dilated. CN IV is involved (the conjunctival blood vessel OS does not intort on attempted downgaze).*

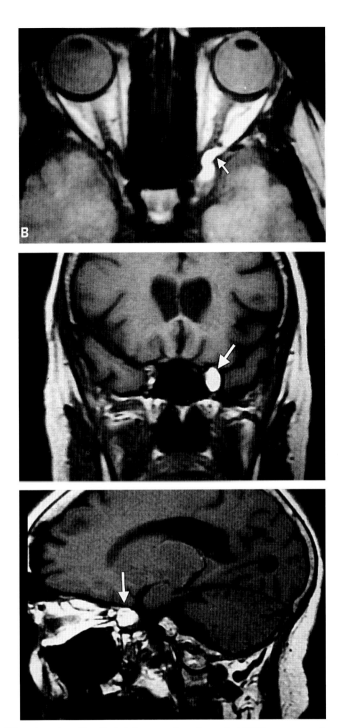

Figure 10–22. *(continued)* **B.** *Axial, coronal, and saggital MRI scans reveal a mass with the characteristics of hemorrhage in the cavernous sinus* (arrows).

INTERNUCLEAR OPHTHALMOPLEGIA

The medial longitudinal fasciculus (MLF), a tract that extends from the pons to the mesencephalon, links the nucleus of CN VI to the contralateral medial rectus subnucleus of CN III to produce conjugate eye movements. The MLF also contains fibers that connect the vestibular nuclei with the ocular motor nuclei. A lesion in the MLF will produce an ocular motility disturbance termed an internuclear ophthalmoplegia (INO).

Etiology

Any disease process that involves the MLF can produce an INO. However, the two most frequent causes of this eye movement abnormality are multiple sclerosis and stroke.

Clinical Characteristics

Symptoms

Patients with INOs do not usually appreciate diplopia. They may complain of a vague visual disturbance that is difficult for them to define. Patients who do appreciate diplopia have the double vision on the basis of an associated neurologic finding, for example, a skew deviation.

Signs

1. Adduction paresis and contralateral abducting nystagmus: the typical picture of an INO is an adduction defect in one or both eyes (resembling an isolated medial rectus paresis) associated with disassociated abduction nystagmus in the abducting eye. If the adduction deficit is complete, this is termed an internuclear ophthalmo*plegia* (Figure 10–23). If it is incomplete, it is called an internuclear ophthalmo*paresis* (Figure 10–24). The side of the INO is named for the side of the adduction deficit. Therefore, a right INO will have a right adduction deficit and nystagmus of the abducting left eye. Rarely, a patient may not have a deficit of adduction, but will have only a slowing of the saccadic velocity in the adducting eye, an adduction lag. This is shown by having the patient look from abduction to primary position and noting that there is a marked slowing of the medial rectus saccade. The eye appears to float inward instead of crisply coming to the midline.
2. Convergence may be intact or impaired.
3. Skew deviation: commonly occurs with unilateral INO and rarely with a bilateral INO. The hypertropic eye is usually on the side of the lesion.

Investigations

The presence of an INO indicates a brainstem lesion; therefore, MRI scanning should be performed. It is not unusual for MRI scans to be normal in the presence of an INO. At times, however, the causative lesions may be evident on neuroimaging (Figure 10–25).

Treatment

There is no treatment specifically for the INO. Patients are treated depending on the underlying cause of the INO. Multiple sclerosis routinely occurs in younger patients and produces bilateral INOs (Figure 10–26). These often resolve. Older patients have INOs on the basis of stroke, and these tend to be unilateral. These also may resolve spontaneously.

Special Forms of Internuclear Ophthalmoplegia

Wall-Eyed Bilateral Internuclear Ophthalmoplegia Wall-eyed bilateral internuclear

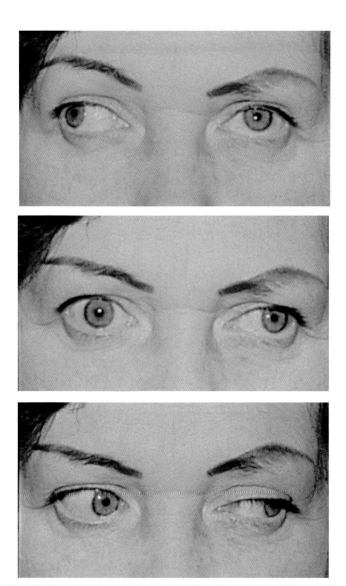

Figure 10–23. *Unilateral left internuclear ophthalmoplegia with inability to adduct the left eye past the midline. There is an exotropia in primary gaze.*

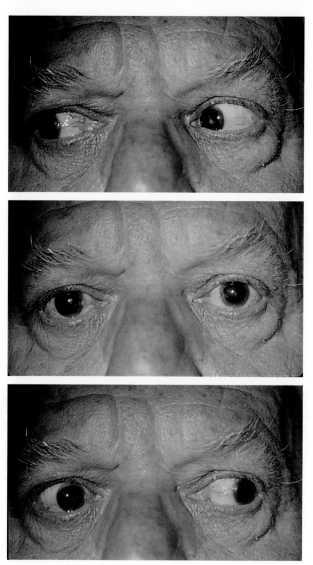

Figure 10–24. *No ocular misalignment in primary gaze. Right gaze is full, but there is a small right adduction deficit on left gaze.*

ophthalmoplegia (WEBINO) is a bilateral internuclear ophthalmoplegia due to a lesion in the mesencephalon. These patients are exotropic (Figure 10–27); whereas most patients with an INO (even bilateral INOs) are orthotropic in primary position. The causes of the WEBINO syndrome are identical to those of INO.

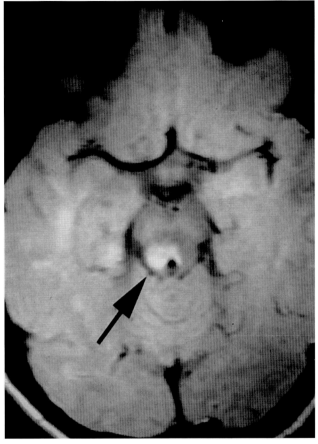

Figure 10–25.   *Axial MRI shows demyelinating lesion (arrow) in a patient with an internuclear ophthalmoplegia.*

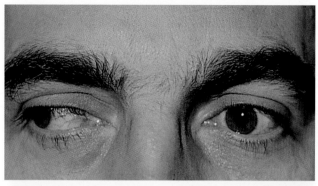
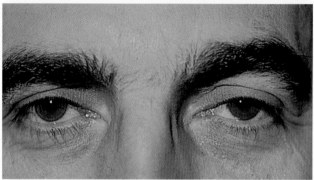
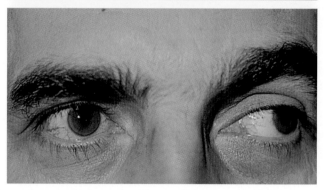

Figure 10–26. *Bilateral INO, but the eyes are straight in primary gaze.*

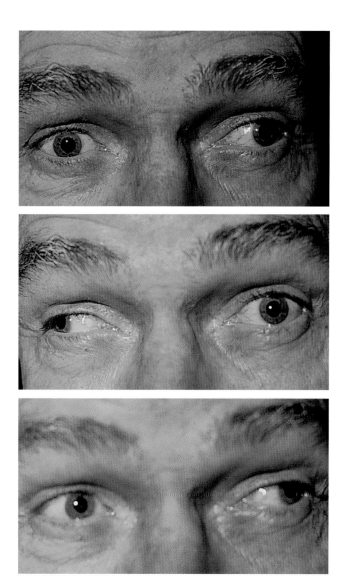

Figure 10–27. *There is an exotropia in primary position (top) with decreased adduction on right (middle) and left (bottom) gaze.*

GAZE PALSIES

Complete inability to move the eyes into right or left gaze is called a gaze palsy, whereas incomplete or limited horizontal excursions are termed gaze pareses.

Gaze palsies may be caused by lesions in several sites. The most common are:

1. Frontal lobe
2. Pontine paramedian reticular formation (PPRF)
3. Abducens nucleus

Frontal Lobe

Cortical lesions acutely may produce a gaze deviation toward the side of the involved hemisphere and a gaze palsy toward the intact hemisphere. This deviation, unlike those of brainstem origin, may be overcome with oculocephalic movements. The gaze deviation and preference usually resolve within 1 week. Ophthalmologists rarely see these patients because they have neurologic deficits, including alteration of levels of consciousness that require hospitalization often in an ICU.

Pontine Paramedian Reticular Formation

The pontine paramedian reticular formation (PPRF) is located rostral to the CN VI nucleus within the pons. A lesion in the PPRF will produce an ipsilateral conjugate horizontal gaze palsy. The eyes may be deviated to the side opposite the acute lesion. Vestibular stimuli may produce ocular deviation to the side of the palsy if the lesion spares the CN VI nucleus and its vestibular connections.

Abducens Nucleus

Lesions of the nucleus of CN VI will also produce a gaze palsy because the nucleus contains, in addition to abducens neurons, interneurons destined for the medial rectus subnucleus of the contralateral CN III. Therefore, a lesion in the right CN VI nucleus will produce a right gaze palsy and not a right CN VI palsy. The causes of gaze palsies are the same as for INO (see p. 186).

Etiology

The most frequent causes of gaze palsies are the following.

1. Multiple sclerosis
2. Stroke
3. Wernicke's encephalopathy
4. Infectious or inflammatory meningoencephalitis
5. Tumors or other mass lesions
6. Degenerative disorders (see PSP)

Clinical Characteristics

Symptoms

Patients with gaze palsies of brainstem origin are asymptomatic unless they have other signs such as a skew deviation, which produces double vision.

Signs

1. Decreased or absent conjugate eye movement to either the right or left or both (Figure 10–28). The gaze palsy is ipsilateral to the side of the lesion, for example, a lesion in the right PPRF produces a right gaze palsy. Oculocephalic movements will produce horizontal gaze in patients with le-

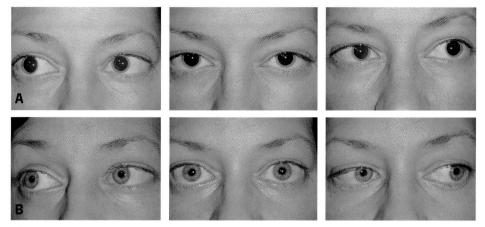

Figure 10–28. *A. The patient has no ocular misalignment in primary position. Gaze to right and left is incomplete. The pupils are dilated pharmacologically. B. Spinal tap was consistent with viral meningoencephalitic process. No treatment was given. Six weeks later, primary gaze is unchanged. Right and left gazes have improved.*

sions of the PPRF, but will fail to produce horizontal eye movements in a patient whose gaze palsy is due to a lesion of the CN VI nucleus.

2. Ipsilateral CN VII palsies are often associated with lesions in the CN VI nuclear area.

Special Forms of Gaze Palsies

Lesions in this area may produce a combination of unilateral gaze palsy and an INO. Such a patient will have an inability to look to one side with either eye (gaze palsy), and on attempted gaze to the opposite side, will have intact abduction, but no adduction. Therefore, of the four possible horizontal eye movements that may be made with the two eyes, only one is possible. Because of this, the syndrome is referred to as the *one and a half* syndrome. This has the same localizing value as an INO or a gaze palsy. The causes of this syndrome are likewise identical to those of an INO and gaze palsy.

Some patients with a one and a half syndrome have an exotropia. This combination is referred to as a *pontine paralytic exotropia* (Figure 10–29).

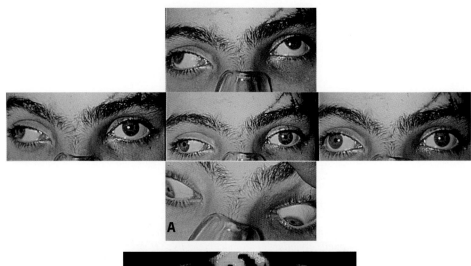

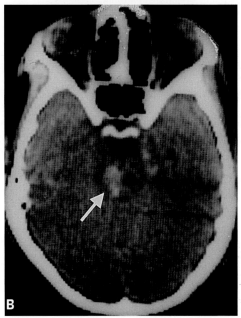

Figure 10–29. *A. There is a large exotropia in primary gaze with a left internuclear ophthalmoplegia on right gaze and complete inability to move either eye to the left. B. CT scan without contrast shows a brainstem hemorrhage* (arrow).

CHRONIC PROGRESSIVE EXTERNAL OPHTHALMOPLEGIA

The disorders collectively known as the chronic progressive external ophthalmoplegias (CPEO) comprise a group of ocular motility disorders called mitochondrial myopathies or cytopathies.

The two forms of mitochondrial myopathy that are most likely to be encountered by the ophthalmologist are:

1. Chronic progressive external ophthalmoplegia (CPEO)
2. Kearns-Sayre syndrome (KSS)

Etiology

These disorders are due to mutations in mitochondrial DNA. These mitochondrial abnormalities lead to decreased protein syntheses and structural abnormalities in the muscle, which on skeletal muscle biopsy appear as *ragged red fibers.*

Inheritance

The CPEOs are caused by mutations (usually deletions) in mitochondrial DNA. Many instances of CPEO are sporadic, but some are maternally transmitted. This means that the mutation may only be transmitted to future generations through the female line.

CHRONIC PROGRESSIVE EXTERNAL OPHTHALMOPLEGIA (CPEO)

This is the most frequently encountered mitochondrial myopathy.

Clinical Characteristics

Symptoms

1. Droopy lid: this is a slowly progressive process that is almost always bilateral. The ptosis usually precedes the other ocular manifestations of this disorder. Ptosis may progress to the point where the lids cover the pupils producing a severe visual deficit.
2. Double vision: usually, there is no diplopia (because the ocular motor defects are symmetrical and slowly progressive). Patients are unaware of the problem until it is pointed out to them during their evaluation for ptosis, or until their eyes become almost completely immobile causing interference with their peripheral vision. These patients often have to move their heads to see to the left and the right. Downgaze is better preserved in these patients relative to the other directions of gaze.
3. Weakness of other muscles may or may not be present.

Signs (Figure 10–30)

1. Ptosis is usually bilateral and symmetrical
2. Ophthalmoplegia is bilateral, symmetrical, and often complete
3. Pupils are normal
4. Weakness of orbicularis oculi or limb and facial muscles

KEARNS-SAYRE SYNDROME

Kearns-Sayre syndrome, a special form of CPEO, develops exclusively in young patients (onset before the age of 20 years). Kearns-Sayre syndrome is defined by the combination of:

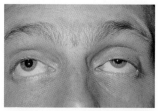

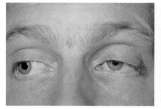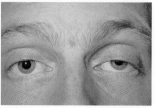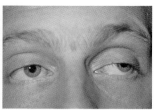

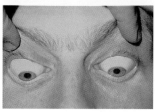

Figure 10–30. *Ptosis is prominent, with mildly depressed ductions in all directions. Downgaze is relatively preserved; upgaze is most affected.*

1. CPEO: (Figure 10–31A) development of the eye movement and lid anomalies are similar to those seen in other forms of CPEO except they develop at a much younger age (usually before 20 years of age).
2. Pigmentary retinopathy: while originally described as atypical retinitis pigmentosa (RP), this pigment retinopathy has a more salt and pepper appearance and resembles more closely the retinopathy of measles (Figure 10–31B). Also in contrast to RP, which normally involves the mid-peripheral and peripheral retina, the pigmentary retinopathy of KSS initially involves the posterior fundus. Furthermore, pallor of the optic disc and attenuation of blood vessels rarely occur in KSS. It does not usually produce severe visual loss, although visual field abnormalities may be plotted. The pigmentary retinopathy may develop before the CPEO.
3. Complete heart block is often the fatal event in these patients. Patients diagnosed

with the KSS should be under the care of a cardiologist. If heart block is not present, continued monitoring should be performed since the heart block may develop at any time during the course of the disease.

In addition, these patients may develop one or more of the following.

1. Cerebellar ataxia
2. Short stature, with delayed sexual maturity
3. Deafness
4. Dementia
5. Endocrine abnormalities (hypoparathyroidism)
6. CSF protein > 1mg/mL

Investigations and Treatment

There is no known treatment for CPEO or KSS. However, KSS patients should be investigated with an ECG, and regular cardiac, neurologic, and endocrinologic assessments.

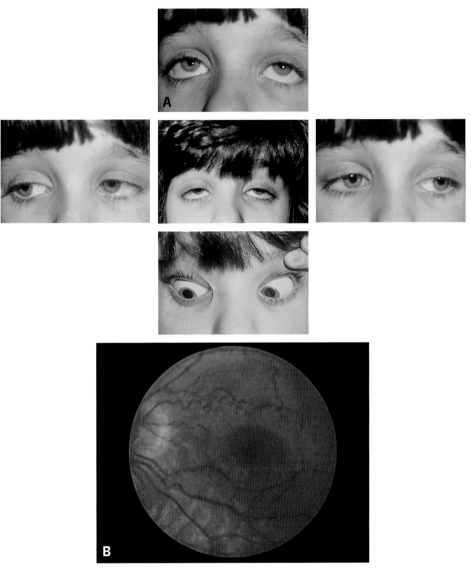

Figure 10–31. *A. Ptosis is marked in primary gaze of this 10-year-old girl. Ductions are mildly limited bilaterally.* ***B.*** *Posterior pole shows typical pigmentary changes associated with KSS.*

PROGRESSIVE SUPRANUCLEAR PALSY

Progressive supranuclear palsy is a neurodegenerative disease characterized by slowing of mentation, disturbances of tone and posture, and limitation of voluntary eye movements.

Etiology

This is a supranuclear disorder of unknown cause that affects predominantly the brainstem reticular formation and the ocular motor nuclei. It usually occurs later in life and is slowly progressive and is usually fatal within 10 years.

Clinical Characteristics

Symptoms

The patient usually has no ocular symptoms or may complain of difficulties because of poor downward vision, for example, seeing their food, walking off the curb or down the stairs.

Signs

1. Slowing of the vertical saccades is the first sign.
2. Impairment of vertical gaze. Usually, downward gaze is affected earlier and more severely (Figure 10–32).
3. Horizontal eye movements are affected late and usually not to the same extent as vertical gaze.
4. Loss of Bell's phenomenon.
5. Intact vestibular ocular response, except that *axial rigidity,* which is characteristic of PSP, often makes testing this difficult.

6. Eyelid disturbances may occur and include apraxia of lid opening or blepharospasm.
7. Other neuroophthalmic signs including square-wave jerks, impaired vergence eye movements, and abnormal ocular pursuit.

Clinical Course

Nonophthalmic Signs

1. Axial and particularly nuchal rigidity.
2. Impaired swallowing and speech.
3. Terminal event is usually aspiration pneumonia.

Differential Diagnosis

1. Parkinson's disease
2. Whipple's disease
3. Multiple infarcts
4. Hydrocephalus

Treatment

There is no specific therapy for the eye movement disorder of PSP.

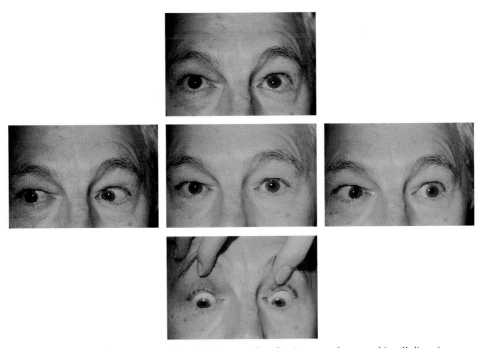

Figure 10–32. *There is no ocular misalignment but ductions are decreased in all directions, especially upgaze.*

GUILLAIN-BARRÉ SYNDROME

The Guillain-Barré syndrome (GBS) is an acute inflammatory demyelinating polyneuropathy that often has neuroophthalmologic signs and symptoms.

Etiology

This disorder is usually seen after a bacterial or viral infection. The most frequent bacterial agent associated with GBS is *Campylobacter jejuni*.

Clinical Characteristics

Symptoms

Patients usually develop symmetrical muscle weakness that progresses relatively rapidly. There is usually a mild respiratory or gastrointestinal illness or a history of vaccinations 1 to 3 weeks prior to the onset of weakness.

The diagnosis of GBS requires the presence of:

1. Progressive motor weakness of more than one limb
2. Areflexia (or hyporeflexia)

Signs

The ophthalmologic and neuroophthalmologic features of the disorder are (Figure 10–33):

1. Ophthalmoplegia: may be partial or total. The most commonly affected nerve is CN VI.
2. Ptosis: is usually present when the patient has opthalmoplegia. It would be unusual for ptosis to occur in the absence of an eye movement disorder.
3. Pupils: GBS may be associated with internal ophthalmoplegia with the pupils being sluggishly reactive or non-reactive to light.
4. Optic nerve anomalies in the form of *optic neuritis* or *papilledema* due to increased intracranial pressure.

Investigations

1. Electrophysiologic testing shows slowing or blocking of nerve conduction on nerve conduction studies.
2. Lumbar puncture shows albuminocytologic disassociation, with a high protein and a normal cellular composition in the CSF.

Treatment

The treatment is supportive. This is usually a self-limiting disease, which recovers completely. Systemic corticosteroids, plasmapheresis, and the administration of intravenous immune globulin (IVIg) have been advocated by some and may shorten the course of the disorder.

MILLER FISHER SYNDROME

A particular subgroup of patients with GBS may be seen more frequently by the ophthalmologist because of the predominance of signs and symptoms localized to the visual system.

The triad that characterizes this subgroup of GBS is:

1. Ophthalmoplegia
2. Ataxia
3. Areflexia

The *ophthalmoplegia* can be identical to that of GBS. In both the GBS and the Miller Fisher syndromes, patients with ophthalmoplegia are found to have an elevated level of anti-GQ1b IgG antibodies.

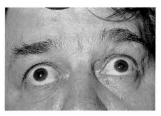

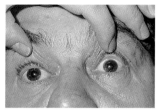
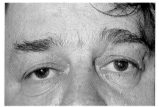
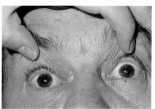

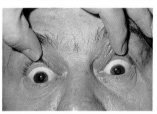

Figure 10–33. *Patient has bilateral ptosis and mid-dilated, poorly reactive pupils. Gaze is limited bilaterally in all directions. The eye movement and pupillary reactions returned to normal.*

Investigations

The CSF findings are usually identical to those of GBS. In addition, MRI scanning is usually normal, however, there may be instances of increased abnormal enhancement of the cranial nerves.

Treatment

There is no treatment for the Miller Fisher syndrome.

The prognosis for recovery is excellent.

MYASTHENIA GRAVIS

Myasthenia gravis is an autoimmune disease that causes weakness in the voluntary muscles.

Etiology and Pathogenesis

The acetylcholine receptor at the neuromuscular junction is essential for the transmission of the nerve signal to the muscle. Myasthenia gravis results when antibodies bind to these receptor sites rendering them unavailable. These anti-acetylcholine receptor antibodies are the immediate cause of MG.

Clinical Characteristics

The basic characteristics of the muscle weakness in MG are *variability* and *fatigability*.

Symptoms

Ophthalmic symptoms include the following.

1. Drooping eyelids are eventually experienced by almost all myathenic patients. It is the initial symptom in approximately 50% of patients with MG. The ptosis is absent or less upon awakening but progresses as the day goes on and the patient tires. It may involve one or both lids and is usually asymmetric. At times, the lids may be completely ptotic to the point where the patient must manually elevate them to see.
2. Double vision: the diplopia of MG also worsens with prolonged effort or as the day wears on.

Nonophthalmic complaints include:

1. Weakness in one or more muscle group, for example, proximal limb muscles, resulting in difficulty walking or getting up from a chair.
2. Pharyngeal muscles: patients may note a change in their voice, which may take on a nasal quality.

3. Difficulty swallowing or breathing constitute a medical emergency for any patient with MG.

Signs

1. Ptosis. There are several characteristics of the ptosis in MG.
   - The lid droop may be accentuated by having the patient maintain upgaze for 2 minutes (Figure 10–34).
   - Manually elevating the more ptotic lid will result in the other lid becoming noticeably more ptotic (Figure 10–35). This is termed *enhanced ptosis*.
   - When MG patients look from downgaze to primary position, the lids will often overshoot and then come to rest in their customary position. This phenomenon is the *Cogan's sign*. However, intermittent lid twitching may be seen in these patients independent of Cogan's sign.
2. Ocular misalignment and decreased ocular motility: myasthenia gravis may manifest any ocular motility disturbance. Diplopia is usually, but not invariably, present. The more frequently encountered abnormal ocular motility patterns include:
   - Upgaze paresis: difficulty in elevating either eye is often seen, especially when ptosis is present.
   - Pseudo INO: there is defective adduction of one or both eyes simulating the INO of brainstem disease (Figure 10–36).
   - Ophthalmoplegia: the eyes become virtually immobile in all directions of gaze (Figure 10–37),
   - Simulating CN palsies (Figure 10–38).
3. Saccades:
   - May show slow velocity with fatigue
   - May have abnormal rapid dart-like saccades ("quiver" or lightning eye movements)

4. Lid weakness: the eyelids are easily opened during forced lid closure indicating orbicularis muscle weakness.

Investigations

Office tests for MG include the following.

1. *Tensilon test:* the intravenous injection of edrophonium chloride (Tensilon) causes the reversal of lid and ocular motility signs in MG in a majority of patients. The patient will revert to baseline in approximately 2 minutes.
2. *Ice test:* ice is placed over the closed ptotic lid for 2 minutes. Myasthenic ptosis will be greatly improved; whereas ptosis from other causes will not (Figure 10–39). Ocular motility limitations will improve after 5 minutes of ice application.
3. *Rest test:* the patient keeps his or her eyes closed for 20 minutes and the ptosis improves.

Laboratory tests include:

1. Acetylcholine receptor antibody assay. The detection of an elevated titer of these block-ing antibodies is virtually diagnostic of MG. Approximately 30 to 50% of patients with ocular myasthenia will have an elevated antibody titer.
2. Electromyography (EMG) reveals a decremental response to repetitive stimulation of affected muscles. The single-fiber EMG may be diagnostic of MG when the routine EMG is not.
3. Chest imaging to detect thymic enlargement or thymoma is performed in all patients diagnosed with MG.
4. Thyroid function studies are performed since there is an increased incidence of dysthyroidism in patients with MG.

Treatment

The therapy options for MG include cholinesterase inhibitors, corticosteroid or other immunosuppressive therapy, thymectomy, and plasmapheresis.

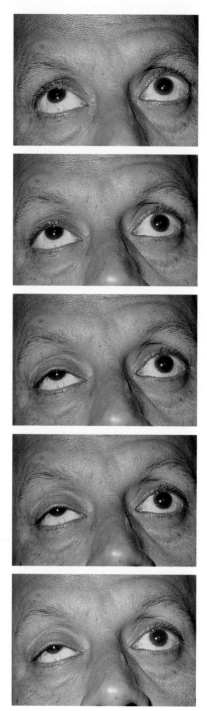

Figure 10–34. *Right upper lid ptosis gradually worsens with sustained upgaze.*

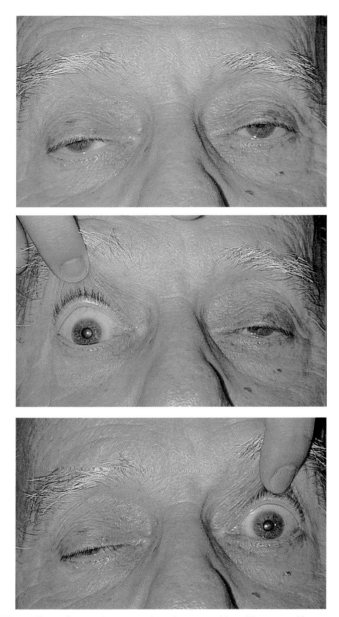

Figure 10–35. *Bilateral ptosis is present in primary position. Note use of brow to try to open the lids. Manually elevating each lid will cause the other to become more ptotic.*

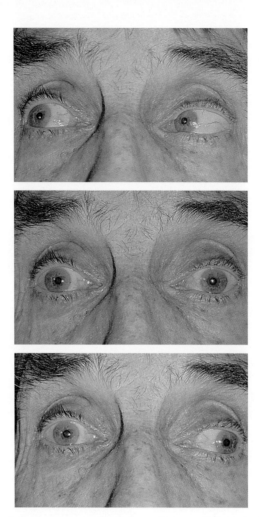

Figure 10–36. *On left gaze (bottom), the right eye does not abduct, simulating a right internuclear ophthalmoplegia of brainstem origin.*

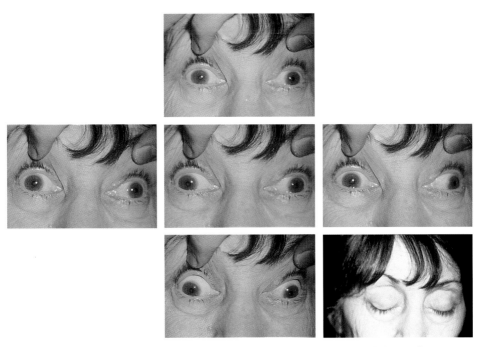

Figure 10–37. *Complete bilateral ptosis and almost complete bilateral ophthalmoplegia resolved completely with oral Mestinon.*

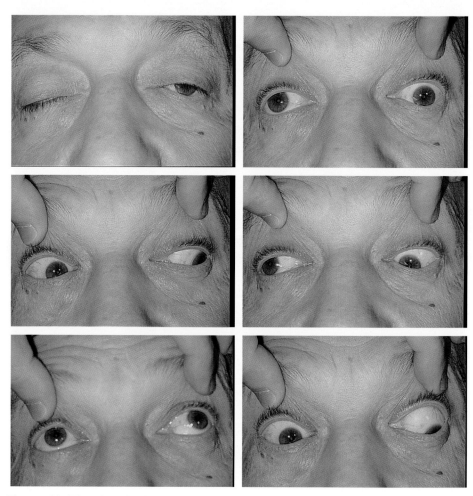

Figure 10–38. *Complete left ptosis (right lid also ptotic). The eyes are exotropic in primary position with decreased adduction, elevation, and depression of the left eye. There is a small adduction deficit OD.*

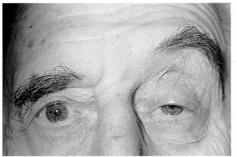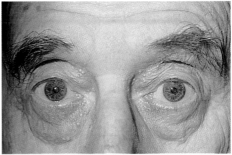

Figure 10–39. *Ptosis on right upper lid (left) improves dramatically following the application of ice to the lid for 2 minutes (right).*

DORSAL MIDBRAIN (PARINAUD'S) SYNDROME

Dorsal midbrain (Parinaud's) syndrome produces a deficit in upward gaze caused by involvement of the vertical gaze centers in the dorsal midbrain.

Etiology

Lesions in the area of the dorsal midbrain that produce Parinaud's syndrome include:

1. Pineal region tumors
2. Hydrocephalus from any cause
3. Trauma
4. Stroke
5. Multiple sclerosis

Clinical Characteristics

Symptoms

1. Diplopia: patients may experience diplopia, but this is due to either an associated skew deviation or unilateral or bilateral CN IV palsies.
2. Transient visual obscurations occur when papilledema is present.

Signs (Figure 10–40)

1. Lid retraction is usually present in primary position.
2. Defective upgaze: patients cannot voluntarily look up, and when attempting to do so, will develop convergence and retraction of the eyes into the orbits (*convergence re-traction nystagmus*). This phenomenon can be elicited by asking the patient to perform an upward saccade or by utilizing downward moving optokinetic targets. This upward gaze paresis is a supranuclear paresis that can be overcome by performing the dolls head maneuver. While the patient cannot elevate the eyes voluntarily, the eyes will go into upgaze when the head is moved into a chin down position while fixation is maintained on a distant target.
3. Pupillary mydriasis: the pupils are usually large, do not react well to light, but their reaction to near response is preserved (light near dissociation).
4. Papilledema: the mass lesions that produce a dorsal midbrain syndrome including hydrocephalus will often produce papilledema.

Investigations

Patients with dorsal midbrain syndrome should have an MRI scan to look for the causative lesion.

Treatment

Treatment depends on the cause of the dorsal midbrain syndrome.

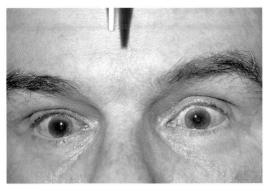

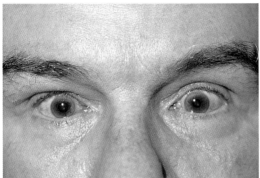

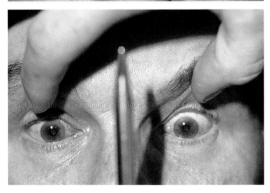

Figure 10–40. *Bilateral lid retraction is seen in primary gaze (middle). Upward saccades cannot be performed (top). The pupils constrict to near (bottom) but not to light stimulus.*

Chapter 11

NYSTAGMUS

Nystagmus is a repetitive oscillation of the eyes that is usually rhythmic. Generally, nystagmus is considered as either jerk or pendular. *Jerk* nystagmus refers to rhythmic back and forth movements in which there is a fast and a slow phase. By convention, nystagmus is described by the direction of the fast phase. *Pendular* nystagmus refers to rhythmic back and forth movements of the eyes in which the velocity is equal in each direction. The nystagmus may be a mixed combination of both jerk and pendular. This chapter is a clinical-based approach to nystagmus and other texts should be consulted for a detailed pathophysiologic understanding of nystagmus.

Nystagmus may cause visual blurring, but usually does not produce other clinical symptoms or signs. Table 11–1 is a list of the clinical characteristics of congenital nystagmus that allow its differentiation from acquired nystagmus. Table 11–2 lists specific forms of nystagmus that can be localized to particular portions of the central nervous system. Table 11–3 lists those eye movements that can be confused with nystagmus.

Several questions can be asked to better determine the nature of the nystagmus.

1. *Is the nystagmus monocular or bilateral?*
   Monocular nystagmus is most frequently seen in the following settings.
   - Internuclear ophthalmoplegia: a dissociated horizontal gaze nystagmus that occurs in the abducting eye contralateral to the side of the MLF lesion (see Chapter 10).
   - Heimann–Bielchowsky phenomenon: long-standing visual loss can lead to low-frequency, monocular vertical pendular or jerk nystagmus in the involved eye. Any condition that causes long-standing unilateral profound visual loss (optic nerve disease, profound amblyopia, dense cataract) may produce this.
   - Spasm nutans: this consists of the triad of *nystagmus* that is usually vertical, dissociated, rapid, unilateral or bilateral, of small amplitude, and pendular; *head nodding* and *torticollis*. It is of unknown etiology and usually starts at 4 to 12 months of age and disappears by the age of 2 years.
   - Superior oblique myokymia is a monocular periodic oscillation.
     —Symptoms: monocular blurring of vision or shimmering of the environment lasting less than 10 seconds, but occurring multiple times a day.
     —Cause: majority have no underlying disease.
     —Looking down or converging may precipitate an attack.
     —Signs: difficult to elicit during examination, but if attack occurs, these are small amplitude irregular intorsional oscillations in one eye.
     —Course: usually resolves spontaneously.

2. *Is the binocular nystagmus physiologic or pathologic?* The forms of physiologic nystagmus are:
   - End-point: this is a fine jerk nystagmus seen in extreme gaze.
   - Optokinetic: this is a jerk nystagmus elicited by a repetitive stimuli moving across the visual field.
     —Slow phase: in the direction of the target movement.
     —Fast phase: opposite direction of target movement.
   - Vestibular nystagmus induced by caloric testing.

—Cold water in ear: produces nystagmus with fast phase in opposite direction to the ear that is being tested.

—Warm water: fast phase in same direction to the ear being tested.

3. *Is the pathologic nystagmus dissociated?* The frequently encountered dissociated nystagmus patterns are:

• Convergence–retraction nystagmus: convergence-like movements associated with retraction of the globe into the orbit. Usually seen with pineal gland tumor or other midbrain abnormality (see page 211, Figure 10–40).

• Seesaw nystagmus: one eye elevates and intorts while the other eye depresses and extorts; the lesion usually involves the optic chiasm or third ventricle, usually in patients with a bitemporal hemianopia.

The forms of nondissociated nystagmus include the following:

A. Upbeat: the fast phase is up and the amplitude is greatest in upgaze. The causes include drugs (phenytoin) or lesions of the brainstem, cerebellar vermis, and posterior fossa.

B. Downbeat: fast phase is downward. This is caused by lesions in the craniocervical junction. This is usually present in the primary position but the amplitude may be so small that it goes unnoticed. It usually obeys Alexander's law (increase in the amplitude when eyes move in direction of fast phase), that is, nystagmus is greatest in downgaze.

C. Congenital nystagmus.

D. Rebound: this is a jerk nystagmus in which the fast phase is in the direction of gaze. However, with sustained gaze, the fast phase changes direction. When gaze is returned to the primary position, the fast phase increases in the direction the eye takes in returning to the primary position. This is caused by lesions of the cerebellum.

E. Periodic alternating: the direction of the fast phase changes in cycles of 60 to 90 seconds.

F. Gaze-evoked.

• Brun's nystagmus: lesions in the cerebellopontine angle may produce a low-frequency, large-amplitude nystagmus when the patient looks to the side of the lesion and a high-frequency, small-amplitude nystagmus when the patient looks in the opposite direction.

• Drug induced.

• Gaze paretic.

G. Vestibular: horizontal jerk nystagmus that may have associated vertigo if it involves the peripheral vestibular system.

H. Latent nystagmus: jerk nystagmus that is absent when both eyes are viewing but appears when one eye is covered. Both eyes beat towards the fixating eye.

TABLE 11–1.　CLINICAL CHARACTERISTICS OF CONGENITAL NYSTAGMUS

Onset at birth or in the immediate perinatal period.
Almost always conjugate and horizontal.
Horizontal nystagmus remains horizontal in vertical gaze.
It is dampened by convergence.
May have a latent component.
There is inversion of the optokinetic reflex.
There may be head oscillations.
Presence of a null point.
Absence of oscillopsia.
It is present during sleep.
Strabismus is common.
Head turns are common.

TABLE 11–2.　LOCALIZATION OF NYSTAGMUS

Nystagmus	Location	Causes
Seesaw	Diencephalon Interstitial nucleus of Cajal or its connections	Parasellar masses, brainstem stroke, septo-optic dysplasia, congenital
Convergence–retraction	Mesencephalon (posterior commisure)	Pineal region tumors
Torsional	Central vestibular connections	Demyelination, infarction (Wallenberg's syndrome), tumors, syringobulbia, arteriovenous malformations
Brun's	Cerebellopontine angle	Acoustic neuroma
Upbeat	Cerebellum	Cerebellar degeneration, demyelination, infarction
Periodic alternating	Cerebellum	Chiari malformation, demyelination, cerebellar degeneration, infarction, cerebellar mass lesions, congenital
Downbeat	Craniocervical junction Cerebellum	Chiari malformation, basilar invagination, cerebellar degeneration, infarction, demyelination, toxic-metabolic

TABLE 11–3. CONDITIONS THAT MIMIC NYSTAGMUS

Condition	Features	Lesion Location
Ocular flutter	Rapid, conjugate, horizontal oscillations	Probably abnormalities of burst neurons
Opsoclonus	Combined horizontal, vertical, and/or torsional oscillations	Probably abnormalities of burst neurons
Ocular bobbing	Rapid downward deviation with a slow drift up to primary position	Pontine dysfunction
Inverse bobbing (ocular dipping)	Slow downward movement, fast upward movement	Nonlocalizing
Oculopalatal myoclonus	Rhythmic oscillations associated with simultaneous contraction of nonocular muscles (palate, tongue)	Interruption of connections in Mollaret triangle: inferior olive, red nucleus, and dentate nucleus

Chapter 12

PUPIL

Anatomy

The pupil receives both sympathetic and parasympathetic innervation. The sympathetic input dilates the pupil and the parasympathetic input constricts it. Therefore, a sympathetic paresis will produce abnormal pupillary miosis while a parasympathetic paresis will cause mydriasis.

Sympathetic System

The sympathetic innervation of the pupil is a three-neuron chain that begins in the hypothalamus with the *first-order neuron* that extends down the spinal cord and synapses at the ciliospinal center of Budge (Figure 12–1). The *second-order neuron* then ascends in the abdomen and thorax coming into contact with the apex of the lung, and in the neck is associated with the carotid artery. At the angle of the jaw, it synapses in the superior cervical ganglion from which the *third-order neuron* originates. The pupillary fibers reenter the skull with the internal carotid artery while the sweat fibers follow the external carotid artery.

Any abnormality along this three-neuron chain produces a clinical syndrome that consists of relative pupillary miosis on the side of the paresis accompanied by ipsilateral upper lid ptosis and lower lid elevation. The lid signs occur because Meuller's muscle in the upper lid and the retractors of the lower lid are sympathetically innervated. When this input is disrupted, the upper lid becomes ptotic and the lower lid rises up (Figure 12–2).

Parasympathetic System

The parasympathetic system (Figure 12–3) begins at the retinal ganglion cells with the fibers destined to innervate the pupil coursing with the visual fibers. The pupillomotor fibers leave this pathway before the lateral geniculate body is reached. The fibers are then fed into the pretectal area and via intercalated neurons the input from each side is mixed and connects to the Edinger–Westphal nuclei. Efferent fibers are incorporated into the CN III and are distributed to the iris sphincter muscle. An abnormality of the efferent parasympathetic input to the iris results in pupillary mydriasis.

Examination Techniques

Examination of the pupil is an integral part of the ophthalmologic examination and should be performed at a minimum on all new patients, but it is reasonable to perform this examination on every patient that is seen in a general ophthalmologic practice. The technique of pupillary examination is as follows.

1. The *pupillary size* of each eye first is determined in a dimly lit room with the patient fixating a distant target. The pupils are diffusely illuminated from below (Figure 12–4A). The pupillary size is examined in bright light by turning on the examination room lights (Figure 12–4B) or by using either a halogen muscle light or indirect ophthalmoscope turned up to its highest brightness level.

2. *Reactivity* of each pupil is tested in a dimly lit room with the patient fixing on a distance target. A bright light is shone in each

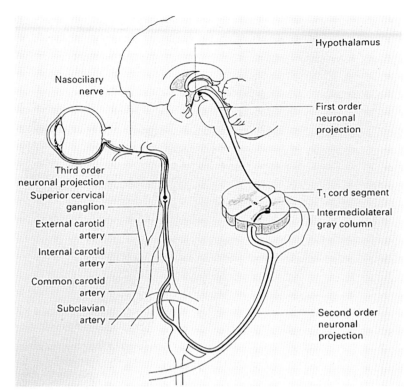

Figure 12–1. *Sympathetic innervation of dilator muscle of iris. Cell bodies of first-order sympathetic neurons in hypothalamus project axons through brainstem to intermediolateral gray column of lower cervical and upper thoracic spinal cord. Second-order neurons project via white rami communicantes through paravetebral sympathetic chain to superior cervical ganglion. On left side, chain in its course splits around subclavian artery. Third-order neurons travel within pericarotid plexus to cavernous sinus, where they join the sixth cranial nerve briefly before entering orbit on first division of trigeminal nerve. These axons enter globe to innervate iris dilator muscle.*

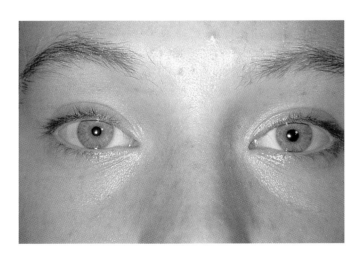

Figure 12–2. *The patient has right upper lid ptosis with the right pupil being smaller than the left.*

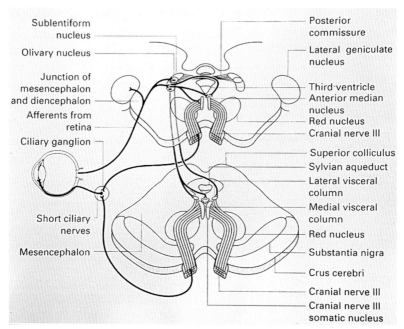

Figure 12–3. *Parasympathetic innervation: pupillary light reflex. Afferents arising in retina project to lateral geniculate nucleus and pretectal (subleniform and olivary) nuclei. Fiber arising from pretectal nuclei project above and below third ventricle and sylvian aqueduct to anterior median nucleus and to medial and lateral visceral columns of Edinger Westphal complex. These nuclei send axons through fasicles of CN III to synapse in ciliary ganglion. Fibers arising from this ganglion project to eye via short ciliary nerves.*

eye and the briskness of the pupillary reactions is recorded (Figure 12–4C and D).

3. The swinging light test is then performed looking for the presence of an RAPD (see Chapter 1).

4. The pupillary *near response* is tested by having the patient fix on a target at 13 in. while the pupils are diffusely illuminated (Figure 12–E). Effort is an important aspect of this test so if convergence does not occur, it is difficult to tell if the problem is pathologic or effort related.

5. Slit-lamp assessment of iris and pharmacologic testing is carried out in specific instances (see sections, Adie's pupil, Mydriasis, Horner's Syndrome).

Pupillary Size

Under normal circumstances, the pupils are equal in size and are within a standard range. Although some people have smaller pupils (particularly older patients) and some have larger pupils (particularly younger, anxious patients), the pupils are usually equal in size. Therefore, anisocoria, that is, a difference in size between the two pupils, must always be suspected of being potentially a pathologic finding. Not all anisocoria, however, is pathologic; *physiologic anisocoria* (Figure 12–5) is seen in approximately 10 to 20% of patients. To determine if anisocoria is physiologic, as opposed to being due to a pathologic process, the pupillary size is

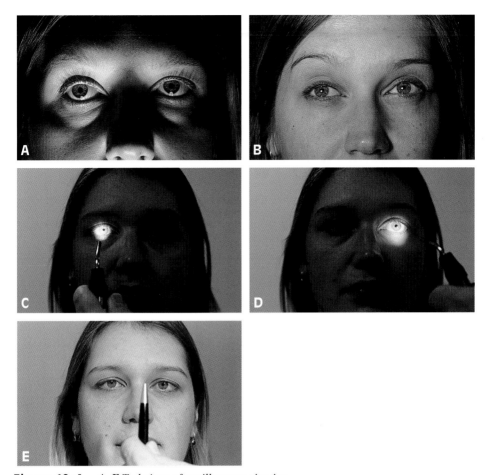

Figure 12–4. *A–E Technique of pupillary examination.*

determined as just described in both bright and dim illumination. In physiologic anisocoria, the pupillary size is relatively the same in both illumination levels. For example, if there is a 30% difference in pupillary size in dim light, a 30% difference also will be present in bright light. Any change in the degree of the anisocoria in bright and dim light indicates pathologic anisocoria (see the following discussion).

Pathologic anisocoria can be due to an abnormality of either the sympathetic or the parasympathetic pathway (see previous discussion). If the anisocoria is greater in dim light, the abnormal pupil is the smaller one and a sympathetic paresis should be suspected. The most likely manifestation of this sympathetic paresis is a Horner's syndrome, which is usually accompanied by ptosis (Figure 12–6).

If the anisocoria is greater in bright light, the abnormal pupil is the larger one, which does not constrict normally. There are a variety of causes of this, including abnormalities in the pupillary parasympathetic innervational system. Adie's pupil and a parasympathetic paresis due to a CN III palsy are the most likely causes of a parasympathetic abnormality. Likewise, pharmacologic blockade of one pupil will produce anisocoria that is greater in bright light (Figure 12–7).

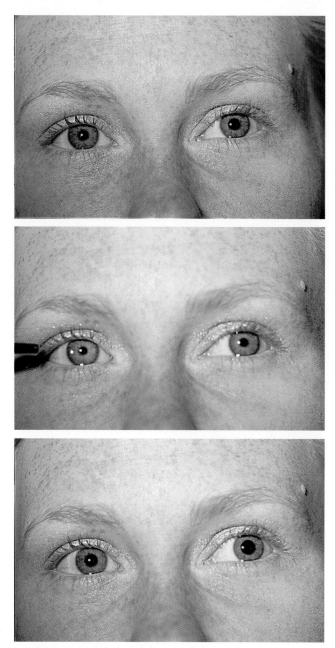

Figure 12–5. *The left pupil is larger than the right in ambient light (top). The degree of aniso-coria is the same in bright (middle) and dim illumination (lower).*

CHAPTER 12   PUPILS

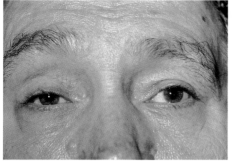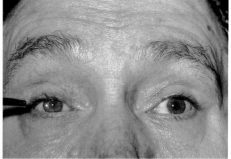

Figure 12–6. *Anisocoria is more prominent in dim illumination, indicating the smaller pupil is abnormal.*

Pearl

In any patient who has anisocoria, it is critical to examine:

1. The lids
2. Ocular motility

This will enable the physician to identify the more important causes of anisocoria, that is, a Horner's syndrome and CN III palsy.

Pharmacologic Testing in Anisocoria

In any pharmacologic testing of the pupil, the testing agent being used should be instilled in both cul du sacs so that the "normal" pupil is used as a control. The most frequently used pharmacologic tests of pupillary function are:

1. Cocaine 10% and hydroxyamphetamine 1% may be used in the investigation of a Horner's syndrome. Cocaine dilates a normal pupil, but does not dilate the small pupil of a sympathetic paresis independent of the anatomic level of the lesion. Hydroxyamphetamine, on the other hand, dilates the normal pupil, and also will dilate pupils with a sympathetic paresis due to lesions of the first- and second-order neurons. However, it will not dilate a pupil with sympathetic paresis on the basis of a third-order (postganglionic) lesion. Therefore, if instillation of cocaine does not dilate the pupil, the presence of a sympathetic paresis is confirmed (see Horner, Figure 12–9, p. 226).

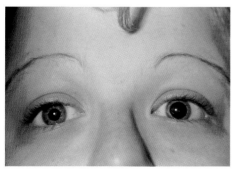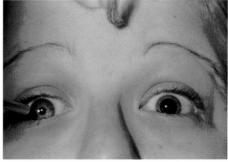

Figure 12–7. *Greater anisocoria in bright illumination indicates that the larger pupil is abnormal.*

If the same pupil does not dilate with hydroxyamphetamine, the sympathetic paresis is at the level of the third-order neuron.

2. Pilocarpine is used in the investigation of abnormally large pupils.
   - Adie's tonic pupil (see page 231, Adie's pupil) manifests denervation hypersensitivity. While the normal pupil does not constrict pilocarpine 1/8 or 1/10 percent, the Adie's pupil will (see p. 233 Figure 12–12C).
   - Mydriasis due to pharmacologic blockade will remain unchanged even when pilocarpine 1% is instilled while the normal fellow pupil will constrict (see p. 230 Figure 12–11).

Reactivity of the Pupil

Even in the presence of isocoria (pupils of equal size), pupillary reactivity should be assessed. The pupils may be abnormal in reactivity and yet be of equal size. Such abnormalities are usually due to parasympathetic disorders and may be seen in processes such as the Guillain-Barré syndrome or botulism. Adie's pupil, which has a tendency to become bilateral, may also produce bilaterally poorly reactive pupils that at times may be isocoric.

Relative Afferent Pupillary Defect

At this point the patient is examined for the presence of a RAPD. The method of examination and its significance is outlined in Chapter 1.

Near Response

Testing for the near response is not performed routinely but is important to document in specific clinical situations, usually to detect light–near dissociation. This pupillary disconnect, where the pupil does not react to light but does to near, is seen in Adie's pupil, Argyll Robertson pupils, and in the dorsal midbrain syndrome among others.

HORNER'S SYNDROME

Horner's syndrome is caused by a decrease in the sympathetic innervation to the eye. The defining signs of the syndrome are *ptosis* and *miosis*.

Anatomy

The sympathetic pathway consists of a three-neuron chain that extends from the hypothalamus, through the brainstem, to the spine, where it first synapses at the *ciliospinal center of Budge* (at the level of C8–T2). It then ascends to come in contact with the apex of the lung and synapses again at the *superior cervical ganglion.* These first two neurons in the chain are referred to collectively as preganglionic. The pathway reenters the skull with the carotid artery. This third-order (postgangionic) neuron, which arises from the superior cervical ganglion, innervates Mueller's muscle of the upper lid and the lid retractor muscles in the lower lid, as well as providing sympathetic innervation to the iris (see (Figure 12–1).

Etiology

Any lesion occurring at any point along this chain will produce the clinical signs of Horner's syndrome.

Clinical Characteristics

Symptoms Often, the patient is asymptomatic or may notice a slight ptosis. Initially, increased accommodation might cause fluctuation of vision. The presence of associated signs or symptoms may assist in localizing the level of the lesion (Table 12–1).

TABLE 12–1. HORNER'S SYNDROME

Level	Associated Signs and Symptoms	Causes	Pharmacologic Test
I	Contralateral hemiparesis Contralateral hemianesthesia Hemihypohydrosis Wallenberg Syndrome Contralateral CN IV palsy Ipsilateral CN VI palsy	Stroke Multiple sclerosis Vetebral artery dissection	None diagnostic
II	Hoarseness Cough Pain in scapula region	Tumors of the lung, breast, and schwannomas Trauma (including surgery) Epidural anesthetic	Hydroxyamphetamine negative
III	Orbital and neck pain Decreased taste Dysphagia Palatal hemianesthesia Headache Involvement of CN III, IV, V, and VI	Carotid artery dissection Neck trauma Tumors and inflam- mation of neck Cluster headache Raeder's paratrigeminal neuralgia Cavernous sinus masses and inflammation	Hydroxyamphetamine positive

Signs (Figure 12–8A)

1. Ptosis of the upper eyelid combined with elevation of the lower lid produce narrowing the interpalpebral fissure and apparent enophthalmos.

2. Anisocoria, with the pupil on the effected side being smaller because of decreased innervation to the iris dilator muscle. The anisocoria is greater in dim light because the pupil with the sympathetic paresis does

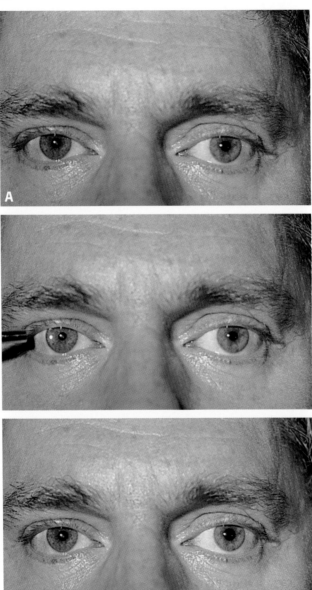

Figure 12–8. *A. A patient with a right Horner's pupil. The anisocoria is greater in dim light. Note that the right lower lid is elevated.*

not dilate normally but the anisocoria is less or disappears completely in bright light. Several factors affect the degree of anisocoria:

- Alertness of the patient: in an alert patient, the normal pupil is dilated, whereas the pupil of Horner's syndrome is less so.
- Resting size of pupils.
- Completeness of the injury and extent of reinnervation.
- Degree of supersensitivity and concentration of circulating adrenergic substance in the blood.

3. Anhidrosis: depending on the site of the lesion, sweat fibers to the ipsilateral face may be involved so that some patients may demonstrate lack of sweating of the forehead. As the postganglionic sudomotor fibers to the face follow the external carotid artery after synapsing in the superior cervical ganglion, a postganglionic lesion may only produce minimal sweat disturbance of the skin of the forehead.

4. Iris heterochromia: if the Horner's syndrome is congenital, iris heterochromia is present with the iris on the affected side being a lighter color than on the nonaffected side.

5. Paradoxical pupillary dilation: denervation supersensitivity leads to a widely dilated pupil with adrenergic stimulation. The pupil on the side of the sympathetic lesion may become the larger pupil as a result of the release of endogenous catecholamines that occurs with intense emotional excitement.

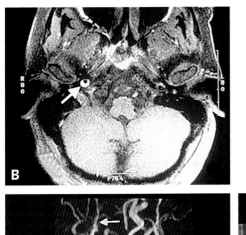

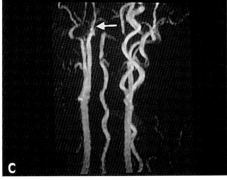
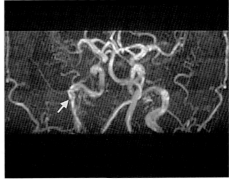

Figure 12–8. *(continued)* **B.** *MRI reveals the characteristic hyperintense halo of blood in the wall of the carotid artery* (arrow). **C.** *MRA (left) shows narrowing and an irregular contour of the internal carotid artery in the neck* (arrow). *The intracranial artery regains it normal caliber and regular contour above the dissection* (arrow) *(right).*

6. Dilation lag: the Horner's pupil initially dilates more slowly in the dark. The anisocoria is more prominent after 5 seconds and decreases at 15 seconds. This effect can be exaggerated by interposing a sudden noise (which increases sympathetic discharge).

7. Skin changes: acutely following sympathetic denervation, the skin temperature on the side of the lesion increases because of loss of sudomotor control and dilation of blood vessels. Hence, there may be conjunctival hyperemia, skin flushing, epiphora, and nasal stuffiness. In the long term, the skin on the affected side may actually be paler. This is because denervation sensitivity of blood vessels results in vasoconstriction.

Investigations

One of the aims of pharmacologic testing is to document the presence of Horner's syndrome, which is done by instilling topical cocaine (2 to 10%). Cocaine dilates a normal pupil by blocking the reuptake of norepinephrine into the sympathetic nerve endings, thus, allowing its prolonged presence to produce mydriasis. Under normal circumstances, there is sufficient norepinephrine constantly present to cause the pupil to dilate. When there is sympathetic denervation, an insufficient quantity of norepinephrine is present at the sympathetic effector cells. Therefore blocking the reuptake does not result in pupillary dilation. Cocaine dilates a normal pupil, but not the pupil with sympathetic paresis. The presence of 0.8mm of postcocaine anisocoria establishes the diagnosis (Figure 12–9). The larger the amount of anisocoria 45 minutes after cocaine instillation, the more secure is the diagnosis of Horner's syndrome.

Hydroxyamphetamine actively releases norepinephrine from the stores in the adrenergic nerve endings, thus, dilating a normal pupil. It also will dilate first- and second-order Horner's pupils, where the norepinephrine is present in the nerve ending of the third-order neuron but is not being released due to the preganglionic sympathetic paresis. With a third-order (postganglionic) lesion, the nerve endings are damaged and there are insufficient stores of norepinephrine to release. Therefore, a Horner's pupil due to a third-order (post-ganglionic) lesion will not dilate.

The combination of these two pharmacologic tests has been used as a basis of deciding which patients with Horner's pupil should undergo further investigation. Since postganglionic lesions tend to be caused by more benign processes, such as migraine, it has been recommended that patients with preganglionic Horner's pupil be investigated, whereas those with an isolated postganglionic Horner's pupil need not be.

However, pharmacologic testing will err in determining the localization of the Horner's lesion about 10% of the time. Therefore, we recommend that all patients with Horner's syndrome undergo MR of the head and neck and CT of the thorax.

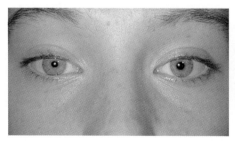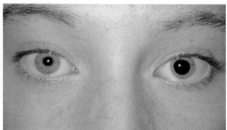

Figure 12–9. *There is ptosis and miosis on the right. After the instillation of cocaine 10% the* left *pupil dilates, but the* right *does not, indicating a* right *Horner's syndrome.*

Treatment

Treatment is directed at the underlying etiology if one is found.

Special Form: Carotid Artery Dissection

This cause of Horner's syndrome also produces pain in the neck, ipsilateral face, or the periorbital area; decreased taste is present in approximately 10% of patients.. The dissection may be spontaneous, caused by minor trauma or by an inherent structural defect of the arterial wall. It may be associated with an underlying connective tissue disorder such as Ehlers-Danlos syndrome type IV, Marfan's syndrome, osteogenesis imperfecta type I, and autosomal dominant polycystic kidney disease.

A subintimal dissection usually results in carotid stenosis or occlusion. A subadventitial dissection may cause an aneurismal dilation of the carotid artery. The diagnosis of carotid dissection may be made on MRI scan alone, where a crescent or circular area of bright signal (blood) is seen within the luminal wall of the carotid artery (see Figure 12–8B). An MRA will show the dissection, usually with marked stenosis or occlusion of the carotid artery (see Figure 12–8C). This testing is sufficient. Catheter angiography need not be performed.

Treatment is aimed at preventing stroke or retinal ischemia and consists of intravenous heparin followed by oral warfarin. The dissections usually heal spontaneously in several months. Repeat MRA will reveal when arterial patency has been restored and the anticoagulation therapy may be discontinued.

MYDRIASIS

Mydriasis is defined as a dilated pupil. It can be unilateral or bilateral. It also can be isolated or associated with other lid or extraocular muscle findings. Isolated pupillary mydriasis occurs in only a few conditions:

Trauma

A dilated pupil can be the result of trauma to the globe. The dilated pupil is usually irregular and pupillary constriction to light is decreased or absent, even in the presence of preserved vision. Both the direct and consensual reaction to light and near stimuli are usually decreased.

Slit lamp examination often reveals rupture of the pupillary sphincter or loss of the sphincter, as evidenced by flattening out of the pupillary collarette. Other anterior segment findings consistent with trauma (eg, a subluxated lens, hyphema, etc) also may be seen (Figure 12–10).

Adie's Tonic Pupil

See page 231.

Pharmacologic Mydriasis

Certain pharmaceuticals produce mydriasis. At times, systemic medications will produce bilat-

eral dilated pupils with reactivity that is usually decreased.

The most frequently encountered clinical condition, however, is that of unilateral mydriasis with a minimally to nonreactive pupil without any lid or ocular motor abnormalities that may suggest a CN III palsy. Topical instillation of a pupillary dilating agent must be considered in this scenario. This may occur accidentally, with the patient being unaware that a pupillary dilating agent has been introduced into the eye.. At times, however, the introduction of the mydriatic agent is purposeful and is done for secondary gain.

The extent of pupillary dilatation with the instillation of mydriatic agents is much greater than the pupil dilation encountered in neurologic conditions, for example CN III palsy. The pharmacologically dilated pupil is usually dilated to approximately 9 mm and does not react to light or near stimulation.

The diagnosis of a pharmacologically dilated pupil is established by obtaining a history, if available, of the instillation of a dilating agent

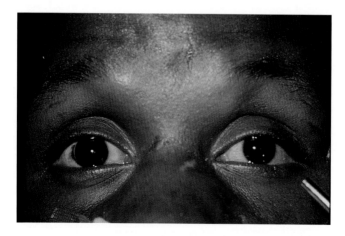

Figure 12–10. *The left pupil is dilated, slightly irregular and does not react to direct light. Note the subconjuctival hemorrhage OD.*

(eg, contamination of the fingers when helping a family member instill mydriatic eye drops or touching the eye after applying a scopolamine patch). If no such history is obtained, proof of the pharmacologic cause of the mydriasis is obtained by instilling pilocarpine 1% into both eyes. This drug will constrict a normal pupil as well as the dilated pupil due to CN III palsy, but will not constrict the pupil that is pharmacologically dilated (Figure 12–11). Failure of the dilated pupil to constrict is prima facia evidence of pharmacologic instillation if the pupillary sphincter is intact. Once this has been demonstrated, no further testing to detect another cause is indicated.

Cranial Nerve III Palsy

It is often suspected that an isolated nonreactive, widely dilated pupil with no other signs of CN III involvement may be due to an aneurysm or mass compressing the interpeduncular portion of the oculomotor nerve. There are few case reports that have documented this association, however, the majority of these patients did not have a truly isolated mydriasis or developed other signs of a CN III palsy within 2 weeks. Therefore, it is far more likely that the cause of a widely dilated nonreactive pupil is direct pharmacologic blockade or an Adie's tonic pupil and not CN III palsy.

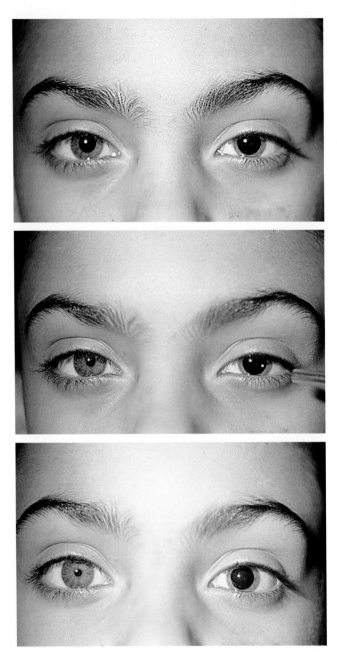

Figure 12–11. *The left pupil is markedly dilated (top) and does not react to direct light (middle). Note consensual constriction of the right pupil. After the institution of pilocarpine 1% (bottom), the right pupil is miotic, the left unchanged.*

CHAPTER 12   PUPILS

ADIE'S (TONIC) PUPIL

This benign pupillary anomaly is characterized by the sudden onset of parasympathetic paralysis resulting in pupillary mydriasis.

Etiology and Epidemiology

This is a disorder predominantly of young women, which appears to occur spontaneously. Patients often notice the anomaly when they look in the mirror, and notice that one pupil is larger than the other. Alternatively, it is noted by co-workers or relatives, who mention it to the patient. Although Adie's tonic pupil occurs in both genders, it is more common in women, with 70% of cases occurring in women and 30% in men. Adie's pupil is unilateral in 80% of cases, with the second eye becoming involved at a rate of approximately 4% per year.

It is thought that this represents a viral infection in the ciliary ganglion. The acute event causes the parasympathetic paresis. The regrowth of the fibers occurs, with misdirection of the accommodative fibers that, because they outnumber the pupillary motor fibers, usurp the latter's actions. Most cases of Adie's tonic pupil are idiopathic. However, Adie's tonic pupil has been associated with herpes zoster, diabetes mellitus, Guillain–Barré syndrome, autonomic neuropathies, orbital trauma (including surgery), and orbital infection.

Clinical Characteristics

Symptoms   Patients may be asymptomatic or may experience:

1. Blurred near vision.
2. A cramping sensation in the eye, which is not usually severe or terribly troublesome.
3. Headache.
4. Photophobia.

Signs   (Figure 12–12A through C)

1. Pupillary mydriasis.
2. Initially, the pupil does not react to light or accommodation.
3. Subsequently, the pupil does not react to light, but reacts slowly and tonically to a near stimulus, then redilates slowly and tonically on refixation at a distance.
4. There is evidence of sectoral pupillary paralysis with loss of the iris collarette (Figure 12–13). There is abnormal movement of the iris to a light stimulus. The portion of the iris with preserved collarette will constrict but the portion where it is absent will not, resulting in a purse string-type movement of the pupil instead of the normally seen concentric constriction. This is often referred to as vermiform movements.
5. Deep tendon hypo- or areflexia (Adie's syndrome).

Certain of these features of Adie's tonic pupil may change over time:

1. The pupils remain large, but over years will become progressively smaller. They continue to react poorly to light and tonically to a near target.
2. Some patients may recover a limited amount of accommodation but still experience a noticeable lag period when shifting fixation between distance and near.
3. Deep tendon reflexes become increasingly hyporeflexic.
4. The other eye becomes involved in approximately 20% of patients.

Investigations and Special Tests

Pharmacologic testing: topical pilocarpine 1/8 or 1/10 % may be instilled into each eye. These

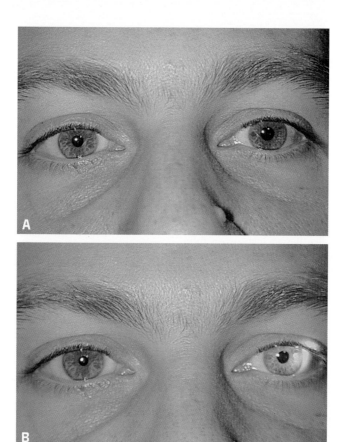

Figure 12–12. *A. The left pupil is larger than the right in ambient light.* ***B.*** *The anisocoria increases in bright illuminations due to poor constriction of left pupil.*

diluted concentrations of pilocarpine will not constrict a normal pupil but will constrict an Adie's pupil because of the presence of denervation hypersensitivity. It should be cautioned that early in the development of Adie's pupil, pilocarpine 1/10% may not cause the Adie's pupil to constrict and will not do so until denervation hypersensitivity occurs (see Figure 12–12D).

Aside from pharmacologic documentation of the unilateral Adie's pupil, no investigations need be conducted, since this is a benign condition. Bilateral Adie's pupils have been associated with syphilis and sarcoidosis, so that the bilateral simultaneous occurrence of Adie's pupil should be investigated for these disorders.

Differential Diagnosis

1. Pharmacologically induced mydriasis
2. CN III palsy
3. Traumatic mydriasis
4. Dorsal midbrain (Parinaud's) syndrome (see p. XX)

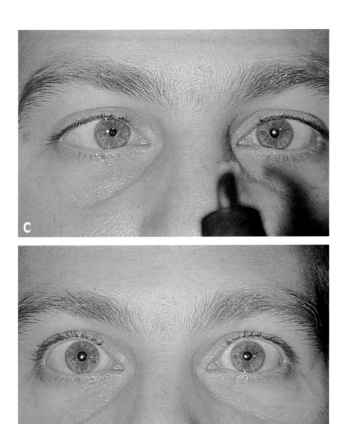

Figure 12–12. (*continued*) *C. Near constriction is slow and tonic, as is redilation where the Adie's pupil may momentarily be smaller than the normal side.* ***D.*** *After instillation of 1/10% pilocarpine, the left pupil constricts while the right does not.*

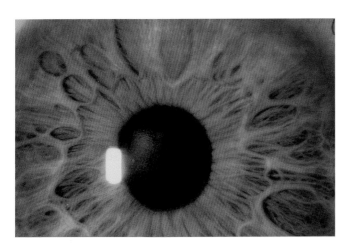

Figure 12–13. *The iris has the ruff partially visible at the 10 o'clock position. The rest of the pupillary ruff is lost and the contour of the pupillary margin is smooth. The normal right iris has an intact pupillary ruff.*

ARGYLL ROBERTSON PUPIL

The Argyll Robertson (AR) pupil is the classic example of so-called pupillary light near dissociation.

Etiology and Pathogenesis

A variety of disorders have been implicated in causing AR pupils. However, most clinicians apply this term only when syphilis is the obvious cause. The exact mechanism by which these patients with syphilis develop AR pupils is unknown.

Clinical Characteristics

Symptoms The pupil abnormality does not produce any direct symptoms.

Signs The following criteria must be met before the diagnosis of AR pupils may be made (Figure 12–14).

1. Vision must be present. Nonspecific light near dissociation will occur with visual loss from any anterior visual pathway cause.
2. Miotic pupils are essential. In particular, in darkness, the pupils are smaller than age-matched controls. During the later stages of syphilis, the pupils may be large and still manifest light near dissociation. These are referred to as *taboparetic pupils*.
3. The pupils show a larger reaction to a near stimulus than to light.

The pupils may also show any of the following characteristics.

1. The abnormality is usually bilateral but at times asymmetric.
2. They may be irregular.
3. Iris atrophy may develop late.
4. The pupils dilate normally to mydriatics until iris atrophy occurs.

Associated findings include the following.

1. Slit lamp examination: interstitial keratitis
2. Dilated fundus examination: chorioretinits, papillitis, uveitis

Investigations

1. Tests for syphilis: FTA-ABS and VDRL
2. Consider lumbar puncture if clinically appropriate (see Chapter XX)

Treatment

The only treatment is directed at the underlying infection if it has not been adequately treated before. The AR pupil remains even after antibiotic therapy is completed.

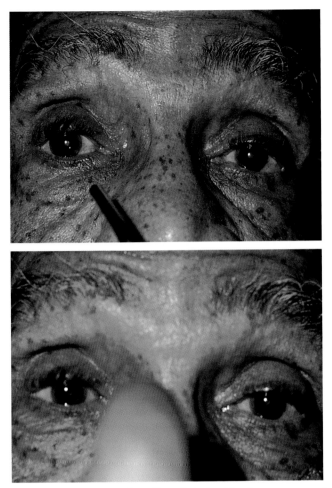

Figure 12-14. *The pupils react poorly to direct light (top) but become more miotic on near testing (bottom).*

Chapter 13

ORBITAL DISEASE OF NEUROOPHTHALMIC SIGNIFICANCE

THYROID-RELATED ORBITOPATHY

Graves' disease is defined as the triad of hyperthyroidism (diffuse thyroid enlargement), orbitopathy, and pretibial myxedema.

Etiology and Epidemiology

It is assumed that TRO is an autoimmune process. However, the exact mechanism by which the changes in the orbit take place remains elusive. Thyroid-related orbitopathy is associated with other autoimmune disorders, such as MG, which is present in 1 to 2% of patients. Orbital findings are due to chronic inflammation and glycosaminoglycan deposition in the soft tissues (extraocular muscles, fat, lacrimal gland) that in turn causes edema and eventual fibrosis. Secondary orbital congestion from decreased venous outflow potentiates the clinical findings.

Incidence

Thyroid disease is common, occurring in about 2% of the general population, with a female preponderance of 6 to 7:1. Orbitopathy is seen to some degree in 30 to 70% of patients with thyroid dysfunction, with the female to male ratio narrowing to 4:1. There is also controversial evidence that patients treated with radioactive iodine rather than medically or surgically for hyperthyroidism may develop TRO more frequently and to a more severe degree. Pretreatment with corticosteroid has been suggested to decrease this problem, but remains unproven.

Although orbital findings usually manifest within 18 months of the thyroid disease, they can either precede or follow the thyroid diagnosis by several years or even decades. Patients are typically hyperthyroid, but may be hypo- or euthyroid. The presence of the characteristic eye disease without any thyroid abnormalities is termed euthyroid Graves' disease. These patients eventually develop thyroid dysfunction in 70% of cases within 2 years of the orbitopathy. Approximately 5 to 25% of patients will present initially to the ophthalmologist without evidence of systemic disease.

Clinical Characteristics

Systemic   Depending on the specific type of thyroid dysfunction (hyper-, hypo-, eu-), initial symptoms include:

1. Weight loss or gain.
2. Increased appetite.
3. Sweating.
4. Heat/cold intolerance.
5. Fatigue.
6. Tremors.
7. Heart palpitations.
8. The thyroid gland may be enlarged.
9. Up to 50% may have a family history of thyroid dysfunction.

Ophthalmic and Orbital   Many patients experience two distinct phases of the disease. Early in the course, the patient presents with symptomatic, inflammatory signs called "active" (Figure 13–1). During this phase, patients have a variety of nonspecific complaints, often misdiagnosed as allergy or dry eye syndrome. As additional orbital inflammation develops, the clinical diagnosis becomes more obvious.

Six months to 3 years later, the progressive changes either arrest or abate, and the patient enters a long-term "inactive" or "burnt-out" phase. At this point, the chance of reentering an inflammatory phase is about 5%. The orbitopathy may present either unilaterally or bilaterally, and may be asymmetric.

Symptoms

1. Lid: a variety of lid abnormalities occur including retraction in primary gaze ("thyroid stare"), edema ("puffy eyelid"), and lagophthalmos (inability to close the eyelids completely).
2. A foreign body sensation, which may be asymmetric, and is either due to proptosis or lid retraction.
3. Double vision is due to infiltration of the extraocular muscles, which become inflamed and subsequently become fibrotic.
4. Loss of vision can be found on the basis of anterior segment disease (corneal exposure and drying) or a compressive optic neuropathy.

Signs

1. Lid retraction is a typical and highly sensitive sign of TRO and is seen mostly in the hyperthyroid state (Figure 13–2A). Upper

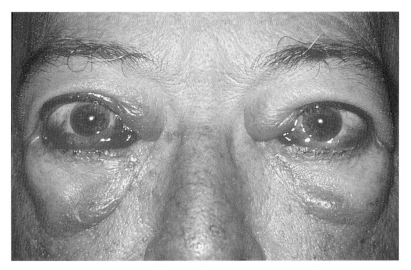

Figure 13–1.   *Acute inflammatory TRO with lid retraction, boggy eyelid edema, conjunctival chemosis, and proptosis.*

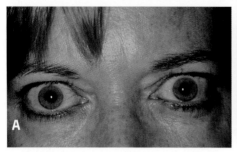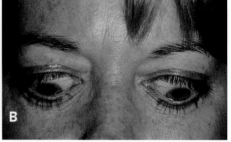

Figure 13–2. *A. Upper eyelid retraction ("thyroid stare"). B. Lid lag in downgaze.*

scleral show should always be considered abnormal and should prompt thyroid function testing. Lid edema may occur in the hyper- or hypothyroid state. The upper lid may lag behind the movement of the globe in downgaze (von Graefe's sign) (Figure 13–2B).

2. Proptosis may be unilateral or bilateral. The most frequent cause of proptosis in adults is TRO.

3. Increased resistance to attempted retropulsion of the globes is found in some patients. Patients with little or no proptosis and increased resistance to retropulsion are at greater risk of developing optic neuropathy.

4. Exposure keratopathy due to lagophthalmos.

5. Ocular injection. Conjunctival injection is most prominent over the horizontal rectus muscle. Conjunctival chemosis is commonly noted inferolaterally (Figure 13–3).

6. Ocular misalignment in any form may occur. However, the muscles most commonly involved are the medial and inferior rectus muscles. Therefore, esotropias and hypotropias are most frequently encountered (Figure 13–4).

7. Increased intraocular pressure, especially in upgaze: this is usually due to restrictive inferior rectus myopathy or a congested orbit (Figure 13–5A). Because this is a mechanical form of increased intraocular pressure, topical antiglaucomatous therapy is often ineffective.

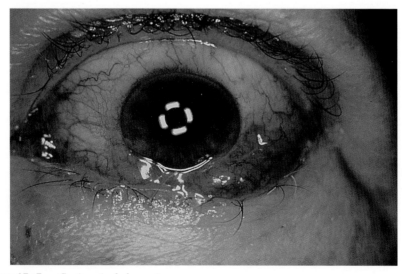

Figure 13–3. *Conjunctival chemosis.*

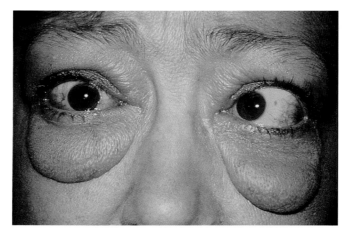

Figure 13–4. *TRO strabismus.*

8. Optic neuropathy of TRO is due to compression of the optic nerve by large indurated muscles at the orbital apex. The clinical risk factors for the development of thyroid related optic neuropathy are:
   • Lack of proptosis
   • Increased resistance to ocular retropulsion
   • Involvement of the medial rectus muscles

Investigations

1. The clinical appearance of the patient with lid retraction is sufficient to establish the diagnosis of TRO (Figure 13–5A). In a typical clinical setting, imaging of the orbit is not required but may reveal enlarged extraocular muscles with sparing of the tendinous insertions. The medial and inferior rectus muscles are most frequently involved (Figure 13–5B). The orbital fat may appear inflamed on MRI and have a diffuse reticular pattern ("dirty fat") on CT.

2. Endocrinologic investigation to detect any thyroid dysfunction should be carried out in patients without a history of thyroid disease. Although a battery of tests is available, in general a selective (sensitive, third generation) TSH is the only screening test needed. This test is especially helpful in patients who are systemically asymptomatic,

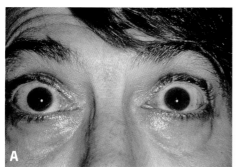
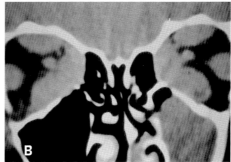

Figure 13–5. *A. Patient on attempted upgaze.* *B. Coronal CT images demonstrate extraocular muscle enlargement.*

since it is effective in detecting subtle degrees of hyperthyroidism.
3. Imaging of the orbit should be performed if the diagnosis is in doubt or in preparation for surgical intervention (see the following discussion).
4. Follow-up schedules depend on the clinical setting. Patients with risk factors for optic neuropathy (see previous discussion) should be examined every 2 to 3 months initially to detect decreasing vision or color perception. Patients with no ocular misalignment and normal retropulsion may be seen every 6 to 12 months.

Differential Diagnosis

A detailed description is found in the section on idiopathic orbital pseudotumor (page ~~207~~ 243, Table 13–1). The same differential diagnosis applies to TRO.

Treatment

General

1. Control the dysthyroid state. Note that control of thyroid function has little effect on the progression of the orbitopathy.
2. Cigarette smoking adversely affects the ocular signs of TRO. All patients with Graves' disease should be advised strongly to stop smoking. The patient should be reminded in no uncertain terms that cessation of tobacco use is important in management of their disease; these conversations should be clearly documented in the medical record.

Specific

1. Systemic corticosteroids: TRO at times will respond to the systemic administration of corticosteroids. Treatment may improve orbital congestion, acute ocular misalignment, and optic neuropathy. Some patients will respond to this treatment, others will not. Prolonged steroid therapy is not indicated because of the risks of long-term steroid use. In the majority of patients, cessation of corticosteroids will result in a recurrence of inflammation.
2. Orbital radiation: there is controversy about the efficacy of orbital radiation. Many reports indicate that it is effective in the treatment of the inflammatory phase of TRO. A recent study indicates that it may not be effective; however, some criticism about the patient selection and duration of the ocular disease keeps the controversy regarding radiation therapy alive. We still employ radiation therapy in select patients with TRO. Orbital radiation is usually given over 10 to 12 sessions (200 cGy each session) for a total dose of 2000 cGy. It should not be repeated because of the risk of additive radiation. It is only indicated in patients who are in the inflammatory phase.
3. Surgery usually progresses in a staged, sequential fashion. Orbital abnormalities are addressed first, followed by strabismus and eyelid repair. Not all patients require each step, but the order is important to maximize predictability of the final result.
   • Orbital decompression is indicated when proptosis must be reduced or when an optic neuropathy occurs. For the relief of proptosis, an anterior decompression may suffice; for the optic neuropathy, a posterior orbital decompression that involves the medial wall of the orbit is usually required. During the inflammatory phase, surgery is reserved for emergent cases of compressive optic neuropathy. Once the inflammation has subsided, surgery is typically safer and more predictable.
   • Extraocular muscle surgery: surgical attempts to realign the eyes should be performed only after the ocular misalignment has been stable for several months (we use 6 months as a minimum).
   • Eyelid surgery is aimed at first correcting upper and lower eyelid retraction and then debulking edematous skin and fat. A variety of techniques are employed, including levator recession, Mullerectomy, and eyelid spacers.

IDIOPATHIC ORBITAL INFLAMMATION (PSEUDOTUMOR)

Idiopathic orbital pseudotumor is an acute inflammation affecting any tissue within the orbit.

Etiology

The etiology is unknown. In the vast majority of cases, there is no associated systemic disease. On occasion, patients with other autoimmune or inflammatory conditions (lupus erythematosus, ulcerative colitis) may present with orbital inflammation. Orbital pseudotumor has no clear predilection for a certain age, gender, or race. No clear seasonal pattern has been proven.

Histopathologically, a mixed cellular inflammatory response is the rule, including neutrophils, lymphocytes, and monocytes, although in some cases (especially children), a preponderance of eosinophils may be seen.

Clinical Characteristics

Symptoms Classically the presentation is acute, with a sudden onset of:

1. Pain
2. Swelling
3. Double vision

Signs Orbital pseudotumor can affect any soft tissue component within the orbit and may manifest signs of:

1. Dacryoadenitis (Figure 13–6).
2. Myositis (Figure 13–7).

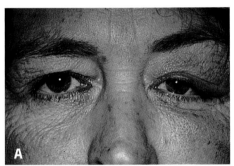
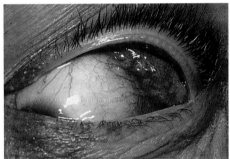
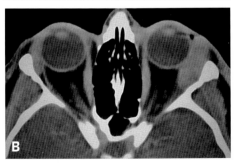

Figure 13–6. *Inflammatory dacryoadenitis.* **A.** *Diffuse injection of the lacrimal gland without purulent discharge.* **B.** *Axial CT shows diffuse enlargement of the lacrimal gland without bone erosion.*

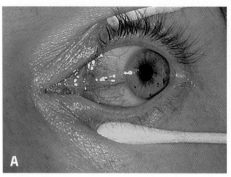
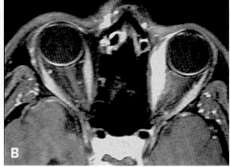

Figure 13–7. *Myositis.* *A. Thickening of the medial rectus muscle insertion with overlying conjunctival injection.* *B. Axial MRI (T1, gadolinium, fat suppression) reveals diffuse enlargement of the muscle, including the insertion.*

3. Optic neuritis.
4. Tenonitis (Figure 13–8).
5. Posterior scleritis
6. Orbital apex syndrome, when the disease affects the posterior orbit.
7. In children, pseudotumor may present with systemic symptoms, including fever, and is more often bilateral than in adults.

Differential Diagnosis

A more complete differential diagnostic list for orbital inflammation is found in Table 13–1. The main entities to consider include:

1. Orbital cellulitis: in some patients, the clinical presentation may be difficult to distinguish from orbital cellulitis. Several findings may be helpful in this regard (Table 13–2). First, orbital pseudotumor tends to present explosively over several hours. Orbital cellulitis typically has prodromal symptoms lasting several days. In orbital cellulitis, the eyelids tend to be tense and deeply erythematous. Conversely, in pseudotumor, there is a softer, pinker swelling of the eyelids referred to as a "boggy edema" (Figure 13–9). Conjunctival edema (chemosis) mirrors this tendency; cases of pseudotumor have a quieter (less injected) chemosis than cases of infectious orbital cellulitis. Furthermore, in most cases of orbital cellulitis, the adjacent paranasal sinuses will be affected with complaints of nasal congestion and purulent rhinorrhea, in contradistinction to pseudotumor, where the sinuses will be clear.

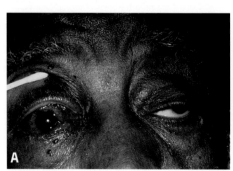
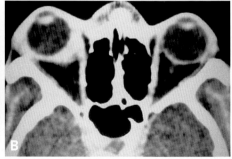

Figure 13–8. *Tenonitis.* *A. Clinical signs of proptosis, external ophthalmoplegia, and conjunctival injection.* *B. On CT, diffuse thickening and enhancement of Tenon's capsule are obvious.*

TABLE 13-1. ETIOLOGIES OF ORBITAL INFLAMMATION

Infectious Inflammation	Noninfectious Inflammation*
By anatomic site of involvement	Thyroid-related orbitopathy
Preseptal cellulitis	Idiopathic orbital inflammation (pseudotumor)
Orbital cellulitis	Reactive lymphoid hyperplasia
Subperiosteal abscess	Granulomatous (sarcoidosis)
Intraorbital abscess	Vasculitic (Wegener's granulomatosis)
Cavernous sinus thrombosis	Polyarteritis nodosa
	Relapsing polychondritis
By infectious agent	Dermatomyositis
Bacterial	Rheumatologic (Sjögren's syndrome)
Fungal	Other (hypersensitivity angiitis, amyloidosis)
Viral	
Parasitic	

* An example of each type of noninfectious inflammation is included in parentheses.

2. Lymphoproliferative disease: the spectrum proceeds from polyclonal, "reactive," lymphoid hyperplasia to monoclonal lymphoma. Orbital pseudotumor should *not* be considered part of this spectrum, since, unlike lymphoid hyperplasia, there is no evidence that pseudotumor progresses to lymphoma. Lymphoproliferative disease commonly presents in an indolent, painless fashion over weeks to months. Additional distinguishing features are found in Table 13–3.

3. Thyroid-related orbitopathy (Graves' disease): a detailed discussion is found in a separate section. Distinguishing features are found in Table 13–4.

4. Adenoviral conjunctivitis presents with preseptal findings. Although initially a unilateral process, autoinoculation of the contralateral eye almost invariably leads to bilateral complaints. Presence of a follicular conjunctivitis along with a tender preauricular lymphadenopathy is diagnostic.

5. Wegener's granulomatosis is a necrotizing vasculitis that may present in either an indolent or explosive fashion. Most patients with Wegener's granulomatosis are male and between 20 to 40 years old. Ocular involvement occurs in 50% of patients. Two variants are seen:
   - Generalized, with involvement of the lungs and kidneys. These patients present with significant, fulminant systemic complaints. A positive c-ANCA serology is the rule and is diagnostic.
   - Localized, with involvement limited to the paranasal sinuses and orbit. Symp-

TABLE 13-2. FEATURES DISTINGUISHING ORBITAL PSEUDOTUMOR FROM CELLULITIS

Features	Orbital Pseudotumor	Orbital Cellulitis
Onset	Abrupt over several hours	Several days
Eyelid	Soft pink coloration, "boggy edema"	Tense, erythematous
CT	Paranasal sinuses uninvolved	Paranasal sinuses involved
Conjunctiva	Variable	Chemosis, injection
Systemic signs	Usually none	Fever, elevated white count

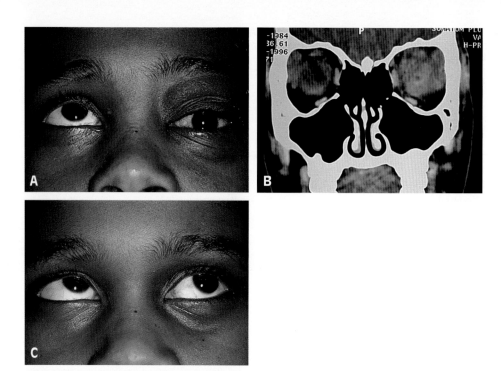

Figure 13–9. *A. Typical pink, boggy eyelids of inflammatory pseudotumor. Note limitation in upgaze. **B.** Coronal CT shows diffuse intraconal enhancement. **C.** Complete clinical resolution 1 week after oral corticosteroids.*

TABLE 13–3. FEATURES DISTINGUISHING IDIOPATHIC ORBITAL INFLAMMATION FROM ORBITAL LYMPHOCYTIC LESIONS

Features	Idiopathic Orbital Inflammation (Pseudotumor)	Orbital Lymphocytic Lesions
Onset	Abrupt	Insidious
Examination	Mimics cellulitis	"Salmon patch" conjunctival mass or orbital mass
CT	Diffuse, poorly defined borders	Molding to orbital structures
Pathology	Polymorphic (mixed cells) Hypocellular Occasional fibrosis	Monomorphic (mostly lymphocytes) Hypercellular Rare fibrosis
Systemic association	Usually none	Lymphoma

TABLE 13–4. FEATURES DISTINGUISHING IDIOPATHIC ORBITAL INFLAMMATION FROM THYROID-RELATED ORBITOPATHY

Features	Idiopathic Orbital Inflammation (Pseudotumor)	Thyroid-Related Orbitopathy
Gender	M = F	F > M
Onset	Usually sudden	Usually gradual
Laterality	Usually unilateral	Usually bilateral
Pain	Yes	Variable
Response to steroids	Rapid	Variable
Imaging (myositis variant):		
Number muscles	~1 (50%)	>1
Muscles	SR, MR	IR > MR > SR > LR
Muscle border	Irregular	Regular
Tendon	Involved (Figure 13–7B)	Spared
Orbital fat	Involved	Relatively clear

Extraocular muscles: SR = superior rectus; MR = medial rectus; IR = inferior rectus; and LR = lateral rectus.

toms are reminiscent of chronic sinusitis. Bone destruction on CT is the rule. Biopsy is necessary for definitive diagnosis, since c-ANCA serology is negative in a significant percentage of patients.

6. Sarcoidosis: periocular or intraocular sarcoidosis may present in either an indolent or fulminant fashion. Involvement of the lacrimal glands is common. History may reveal constitutional symptoms as well as complaints of shortness of breath or a misdiagnosis of asthma. Ocular examination may reveal eyelid and conjunctival nodules, evidence of previous uveitis (keratic precipitates), iris nodules, vitreous debris, and cotton-wool spots. Optic neuritis may occur. Angiotensin converting enzyme (ACE) and chest x-ray may be helpful, but can prove negative in a localized variant known as "orbital sarcoid."

Special Form One rare variant of orbital inflammation, known as sclerosing pseudotumor, is more chronic and causes significant tissue destruction from secondary fibrosis. This form of orbital inflammation is poorly responsive to corticosteroid therapy and may require more drastic measures, including chemotherapeutic agents, repeated surgical debulking, and on occasion, exenteration. The clinical and histopathologic picture is so atypical of classic orbital pseudotumor that some experts have appropriately questioned whether this diagnosis even belongs within the rubric of orbital inflammation.

Investigations

1. CT or MR imaging will reveal a poorly circumscribed, infiltrating enhancement of orbital tissue, and may be limited to specific tissue (muscle, lacrimal gland). Bone destruction is very atypical and necessitates tissue biopsy.
2. On occasion, B-scan ultrasonography is helpful in cases of posterior scleritis, which may not be visible on CT or MRI.
3. Systemic work-up is rarely helpful and is usually not indicated. In patients where differentiation from infection is difficult, a CBC may be obtained. An elevated white count and left shift may be seen in both infectious and noninfectious orbital inflammation. Bacterial infection will usually result in a neutrophilia with left shift, while in some cases of pseudotumor, an eosinophilia may be present.
4. Orbital biopsy is performed in atypical cases, after several recurrences, or with

treatment failure. In Europe, the standard of care appears to mandate an initial tissue diagnosis in all cases of presumed orbital pseudotumor.

5. In cases that present atypically (subacute/chronic, bilaterally in adults) or respond poorly to corticosteroid treatment (recalcitrant or recurrent cases), a lower threshold for a complete systemic work-up and tissue biopsy in search of another cause should be aggressively pursued.

Treatment

1. Corticosteroids. In adults, prednisone 80 to 100 mg daily usually results in rapid and dramatic clinical improvement, often after only one dose; pediatric doses should be calculated based on body weight. Relapses are common and are usually related to a rapid taper of corticosteroids.

2. Nonsteroidal antiinflammatory medications (NSAIDs). In patients who are intolerant of corticosteroids, the initial corticosteroid dose may be tapered more rapidly while a steady dose of NSAIDs is maintained, followed by a slow NSAID taper.

3. Radiation therapy. A course of low-dose (2000 cGy) orbital radiotherapy may be considered. Many experts mandate tissue biopsy before proceeding with radiotherapy.

4. If any doubt is present between orbital pseudotumor and orbital cellulitis, as occurs more often in children than in adults, it is prudent to first begin a trial of intravenous antibiotics with close clinical follow-up. If symptoms fail to improve after 48 hours, a "test dose" of corticosteroids may be given while still maintaining antibiotic coverage. A rapid response to corticosteroids is indicative of a noninfectious inflammation

CAVERNOUS SINUS FISTULAS

Acquired arteriovenous (AV) communications (fistulas) affecting the orbit most commonly occur in the cavernous sinus.

Etiology

Arteriovenous fistulas within the cavernous sinus generally fall into two categories:

1. *High-flow* fistulas are usually the result of trauma, occur in younger patients, and involve an abnormal connection between the carotid siphon and the cavernous sinus venous plexus. The term carotid-cavernous fistula is used interchangeably with high-flow fistula.

2. *Low-flow* fistulas typically occur spontaneously in older patients. The abnormality occurs between one of the small arterial feeders of the lateral dural wall and the venous plexus of the cavernous sinus, hence the term "dural-sinus fistula."

Clinical Characteristics

Symptoms

1. Visual acuity varies from normal to poor.
2. Diplopia.
3. Red eye.
4. Headache may be present.
5. A "whooshing" or "rushing" sound in the head.

Signs

1. Proptosis.
2. External ophthalmoplegia at times with ocular misalignment (Figure 13–10A).
3. Auscultation over the superior orbital rim may reveal a bruit, although this is an admittedly uncommon finding.
4. The conjunctival vessels associated with fistulae are diffusely engorged and tortuous ("arteriolization"). The vascular engorge-ment often extends to the limbus (Figure 13–10B).

5. Intraocular pressure may be elevated. Applanation tonometry often shows a significant pulsatilty to the Myers' prisms.

6. Iris neovascularization may occur from chronic ocular ischemia.

7. A RAPD and dyschromatopsia are present if an optic neuropathy develops.

8. Venous engorgement or central retinal vein occlusion may be seen on funduscopic examination (Figure 13–10C). Exudative retinal or choroidal detachments are less common.

9. Ocular or macular ischemia.

Investigations

1. Orbital color Doppler ultrasonography shows engorgement of the SOV, reversal of flow, and an arterial wave form within the SOV (Figure 13–11). Doppler ultrasonography is highly sensitive in this disorder and should be utilized in all cases to rule in or rule out the diagnosis.

2. An enlarged, S-shaped SOV in the superior orbit, just beneath the superior rectus/levator complex on CT or MRI (Figure 13–12).

3. Selective arteriography is performed if treatment of the fistula is planned (Figure 13–13A).

Treatment

1. In high-flow fistulas that present with severe orbital signs, including progressive optic neuropathy, treatment is indicated. Treatment is performed by neuroradiologic interventionalists. The location of the ab-

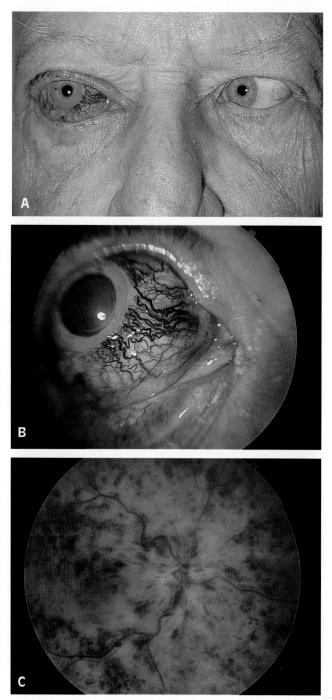

Figure 13–10. *Clinical signs.*   ***A.*** *Mild proptosis and an abduction deficit are noted on the* right.   ***B.*** *Arteriolization of conjunctival vessels.*   ***C.*** *Central retinal vein occlusion.*

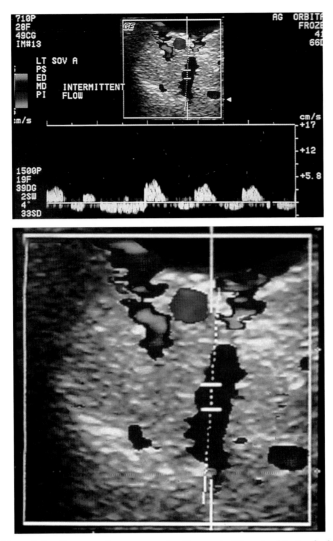

Figure 13–11. *Color Doppler ultrasonography. Reversal of flow (red instead of the usual blue) is noted in the SOV.*

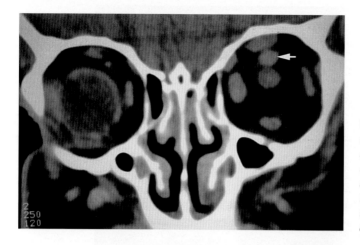

Figure 13–12. *Coronal CT imaging reveals an engorged superior ophthalmic vein* (arrow) *along with diffuse enlargement of the extraocular muscles on the affected side.*

normal connection is delineated using conventional arteriography and, preferably at the same time, the fistula is closed with a variety of techniques, including glue, balloons, or thrombogenic coils (Figure 13–13B). On occasion, the fistula cannot be approached using conventional intraarterial routes. In such cases, the fistula may be closed from an SOV approach utilizing a lid crease incision. The patient is always warned about the potential complications of arteriography, including stroke and death, as well as the risks of fistula closure, including visual loss, worsening of orbital congestion, and neovascularization due to ocular ischemia.

2. In low-flow fistulas no treatment is necessary unless the intraocular pressure is uncontrolled or other symptoms develop, since these fistulas often close spontaneously.

3. A paradoxical worsening of symptoms may be seen in low-flow fistulas. As thrombosis forms in the SOV, the patient may present with a marked increase in signs and symptoms. If possible, conservative management is indicated for 48 to 72 hours, at which time the symptoms should begin to abate as alternate orbital venous drainage forms. If no improvement occurs after this time, the patient should undergo repeat workup to assure that a low-flow state has not converted into a high-flow abnormality.

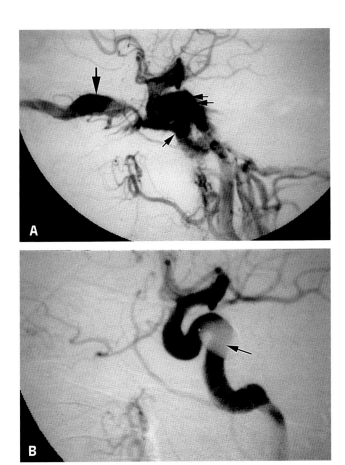

Figure 13-13. *Arteriography.* **A.** *An abnormal connection is noted between the carotid siphon* (small arrow) *and the cavernous sinus* (double arrow), *with secondary engorgement of the SOV* (large arrow). **B.** *Flow into the SOV ceases after placement of a detachable balloon* (arrow) *into the cavernous sinus.*

INDEX

INDEX

Note: Page numbers followed by t *and* f *indicate tables and figures, respectively.*

D

De Morsier's syndrome (septooptic dysplasia), 105
Demyelinating lesions, 15, 21
Demyelinating plaques, 18*f*
Diabetes, 30*f,* 31
Diabetic papillopathy, 63, 64*f*
Diabetic retinopathy, 30*f*
Diffusion-weighted image (DWI), 21–22
  abscess definition of, 22
  demyelinating plaques definition in, 22
  stroke diagnosis with, 22
  tumor definition with, 22
Diplopia, 158*f*
Diplopia evaluation
  binocular single vision visual field for, 149, 151*f*
  comitant or incomitant, 144–145
  ductions and versions for, 146–147
  forced duction test in, 148–149, 150*f,* 151*f*
  lids and pupils in, 149
  monocular, 144
  nystagmus and, 149
  ocular cephalic movements in, 149
  primary and secondary deviation in, 146–147, 147*f*
  prism cover test, 145–146
  red lens or Maddox rod in , 146–147
  saccades and pursuits in, 147–148
Dominant optic atrophy, 92, 93*f,* 94*f*
Dorsal midbrain (Parinaud's) syndrome, 210, 211*f*
  clinical characteristics of, 210
  etiology of, 210
  investigations of, 210
  treatment for, 210

E

Emboli, visible, 28
Endarterectomy, 31
Erythrocyte sedimentation rate (ESR), 59
Esotropia, 166*f,* 167*f,* 168*f,* 170*f,* 173*f,* 174*f,* 175*f*
Exotropia, 178*f,* 187f, 191*f,* 194*f*

F

Farnsworth Munsel 100 hue, *4*
Farnsworth panel D15, *4*
FLAIR (fluid attenuated inversion recovery), 21
Folic acid deficiency, 71

G

Gadolinium, 15, 20
Gaze palsies, 192, 193*f*
  abducens nucleus, 192
  clinical characteristics of, 192–193
  etiology of, 192
  frontal lobe, 192
  pontine paramedian reticular formation, 192
  special forms of, 193
Giant cell arteritis (GCA), 56
  clinical characteristics of, 56–58
    signs of, 57–59
    symptoms of, 56–57
  diagnosis of, 59
  incidence of, 56
  pathogenesis and etiology of, 56
  treatment for, 60
Glioma,
  chiasmal syndrome, 127,129*f*
  malignant, 85, 85*f,* 86*f*
  optic nerve, 80-84
Goldmann manual perimetry, 15
Grave's disease. *See* Thyroid-related orbitopathy
Guillain-Barré syndrome (GBS), 200, 201*f*
  clinic characteristics of, 200
  etiology of, 200
  investigations of, 200
  treatment for, 200

H

Heimann-Bielchowsky phenomenon, 212
Hemihypoplasia (Topless disc syndrome), 104

Lesions
  asymptomatic multiple metastatic, 171*f*
  demyelinating, 15, 21
  macular, 7
  optic disc, 10
  pathological, 21
  retinal, 10
  in retinal pigment epithelium, 45*f*
  retrobulbar prechiasmal optic nerve, 10

M

Magnetic resonance imaging (MRI),
      14–15, 22
  contrast enhancement for, 15, 16*f*–17*f*,
      20
  high-field strength systems, 14, 21
  pulse sequences of, 15, 21
  safety limitations of, 14
  soft tissue accentuation of, 14
  T1WI (T1 weighted image) of, 15,
      16*f*–17*f*
  T2WI (T2 weighted image) of, 15,
      16*f*–17*f*
  weighted image of, 15
Malignant glioma
  clinical characteristics of, 85
  etiology and epidemiology of, 85
  investigations of, 85
  of optic nerve, 85*f,* 86*f*
Medial longitudinal fasciculus (MLF),
      186
Meningioma
  chiasmal syndrome, 127
  clivus, 24*f*
  optic nerve sheath 87, 87*f,* 88*f*
  parasellar 128*f*
  perioptic, 23*f*
  suprasellar meningioma, 119*f*
Metamorphopsia, 5
Methanol
  toxic optic neuropathies of, 71–72, 73*f*
Methylprednisolone, 37*t,* 38*t,* 38*f*
Migraine
  arteriovenous malformation, 141*f*
  classification of, 139

clinical characteristics of, 139
differential diagnosis of, 139
epidemiology of, 139
fortification scotoma, 140*f*
investigations of, 140
treatment for, 141
Miller Fisher syndrome, 200
  investigations of, 201
  treatment for, 201
Mitochondrial myopathies
  etiology of, 195
  inheritance of, 195
Molecular diffusion, 21
Mucormycosis, 31
  non-septate hyphae, 181*f*
Multinucleated giant cells, 60*f*
Multiple cranial nerve palsies, 176
  other causes of, 183
Multiple sclerosis, 15, 19*f,* 32
  clinically definite (CDMS), 36
Myasthenia gravis, 202, 204*f,* 205*f,* 206*f,*
      207f, 208*f,* 209*f*
  clinical characteristics of, 202–203
  etiology and pathogenesis of, 202
  investigations of, 203
  treatment for, 203
Mydriasis
  Adie's tonic pupil, 231
  cranial nerve III palsy, 229
  pharmacologic, 228–229, 230*f*
  trauma, 228, 228*f*

N

Neurofibromatosis type 1
  optic nerve glioma, 82*t*
Neuroophthalmic examination, 2
  efferent system
    diplopia, 144
Neuroretinitis, 41. *See also* Hypertensive
      retinopathy
  clinical characteristics of, 41
  etiology of, 41
  investigations of, 41
  treatment for, 41
Neurosarcoidosis, 119*f,* 133f

Nonarteritic anterior ischemic optic
  neuropathy (NAION), 54–55,
  57
  clinical characteristics of, 54–55
  course of, 55
  diagnosis and investigations of, 55
  pathogenesis and etiology of, 54
  treatment for, 55
Nonphysiologic visual loss
  decreased vision and, 142–143, 143*f*
  no vision and, 142
  visual field loss and, 142–143
Nuclear magnetic resonance spectrometry
  (NMR), 14
Nutritional deficiencies and toxic optic
  neuropathies, 69, 70*f*
  clinical presentation of, 69
  diagnosis of, 69
  differential diagnosis of bilateral visual
    loss and, 70*t*
  etiology and epidemiology of, 69
  treatment for, 69
Nystagmus, 212
  binocular
    end-point, 212
    optokinetic, 212
    vestibular, 212
  clinical characteristics of, 214*t*
  dissociated
    convergence-retraction, 213
    seesaw, 213
  localization of, 214*t*
  mimicking conditions of, 215*t*
  monocular
    Heimann-Bielchowsky phenomenon
      in, 212
    internuclear ophthalmoplegia in,
      212
    spasm nutans in, 212
    superior oblique myokymia in,
      212
  nondissociated
    congenital, 213
    downbeat, 213
    gaze evoked, 213
  latent, 213
  periodic alternating, 213
  rebound, 213
  upbeat, 213
  vestibular, 213

O

Occluder, 3*f*
Ophthalmologic assessment, 2
Ophthalmoplegia, 180*f*, 184
  chronic progressive external
    ophthalmoplegia (CPEO), 195
  internuclear ophthalmoplegia (INO),
    186, 187*f*, 188*f*, 189*f*, 212
  wall-eyed bilateral internuclear ophthal-
    moplegia (WEBINO), 186–189
Ophthalmoscopy, 9
Optic chiasm, 118
  compression of, 18*f*
  demyelinating plaque of, 131*f*
  prolapse of, 130*f*
  radiation necrosis of, 129*f*
  visual field abnormalities in
    bitemporal hemianopia, 118
    homonymous hemianopia, 118, 119*f*
    junction scotoma, 118
Optic disc
  elevated, 54*f*
  with granuloma, 44*f*
  hyperemic, 34*f*
  infarcted, 57*f*
  lesions of, 10
  with nerve fiber layer edema and
    hemorrhage, 42*f*
  at risk, 54*f*
Optic disc colobomas, 107, 108*f*, 108*t*,
    109*f*
  clinical characteristics of, 107
  etiology and epidemiology of, 107
  investigations of, 107
  treatment for, 107
Optic disc drusen, 100*f*, 101*f*, 102*f*, 103*f*
  differential diagnosis of, 99
  epidemiology and etiology of, 99

Syphilitic optic neuropathy, 50
  bilateral papillitis from, 51*f*
  clinical characteristics of, 50
  CSF testing for, 53*t*
  diagnosis of, 52
  etiology of, 50
  ocular manifestations of, 50*t*
  tests for, 52–53*t*
  treatment for, 52

T

Tangent screen, 13
Thiamine deficiency, 71
Thrombosis, venous, 22
Thyroid-related orbitopathy (Grave's
      disease)
  clinical characteristics of
    ophthalmic and orbital, 237, 237*f*
    signs of, 237–239, 238*f,* 239*f*
    symptoms of, 237
    systemic, 236–237
  differential diagnosis of, 240
  etiology and epidemiology of, 236
  incidence of, 236
  investigations of, 239–240, 239*f*
  treatment for
    general, 240
    orbital radiation, 240
    surgery, 240
    systemic corticosteroids, 240
Tissue specific relaxation properties, 15
Tobacco-alcohol amblyopia
  toxic optic neuropathies, 69, 72
Topless disc syndrome (Hemihypoplasia),
      104

Toxic optic neuropathies, 71–72. *See also*
      Nutritional deficiencies
  characteristics of, 71
  clinical presentation of, 71
  ethambutol, 72
  medications producing, 72*t*
  methanol, 71–72, 73*f*
Transient ischemic attacks (TIA), 31
Traumatic optic neuropathy, 113, 114*f,*
      116*f,* 117*f*
  clinical characteristics of, 113, 115
  epidemiology and etiology of, 113
  investigations of, 115
  treatment for, 115
Tumors, 15
  pituitary, 18*f*

V

Vascular malformation, 22
Vasculitis, 28
Visible emboli, 7
Visual acuity, 2
Visual evoked responses (VER), 34
Visual field, 10
  abnormalities in, 33*f*
  extent of, 10
Visual field testing
  confrontation visual fields in,
      10–11
  finger counting in, 11–12*f*
  kinetic manual perimetry in, 13
  static automated perimetry in, 13
  tangent screen in, 13
Vitamin B$_{12}$ deficiency, 71
Vitreous hemorrhages, 7